The treatment of obsessions

Cognitive behaviour therapy: science and practice series

Edited by

David Clark, *Institute of Psychiatry, London, UK*

Christopher Fairburn, *University of Oxford, Oxford, UK*

Steven Hollon, *Vanderbilt University, Nashville, USA*

The treatment of obsessions

S. Rachman

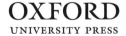
OXFORD
UNIVERSITY PRESS

OXFORD
UNIVERSITY PRESS

Great Clarendon Street, Oxford OX2 6DP

Oxford University Press is a department of the University of Oxford.
It furthers the University's objective of excellence in research,
scholarship, and education by publishing worldwide in

Oxford New York

Auckland Bangkok Buenos Aires Cape Town Chennai
Dar es Salaam Delhi Hong Kong Istanbul Karachi Kolkata
Kuala Lumpur Madrid Melbourne Mexico City Mumbai Nairobi
São Paulo Shanghai Taipei Tokyo Toronto

Oxford is a registered trade mark of Oxford University Press
in the UK and in certain other countries

Published in the United States
by Oxford University Press Inc., New York

© Oxford University Press 2003

The moral rights of the author have been asserted

Database right Oxford University Press (maker)

First published 2003
Reprinted 2004 (twice)

A catalogue record for this book is available from the British Library

Library of Congress Cataloging in Publication Data
(Data available)

ISBN 0 19 851537 5

10 9 8 7 6 5 4 3

Typeset by Integra Software Services Pvt. Ltd, Pondicherry 605 005, India
Printed in Great Britain
on acid-free paper by
Biddles Ltd, King's Lynn, Norfolk

Acknowledgements

Numerous colleagues and students have contributed to the evolution of the theory and the deduced treatment. In particular I wish to thank Professor D.M. Clark, Mr P. de Silva, Professor M. Freeston, Professor P. Salkovskis, Dr R. Shafran, and the colleagues and students who took part in testing and shaping the therapy and background research: Jason Carr, Nichole Fairbrother, Tracey Lindberg, Sarah Newth, Michelle Patterson, Adam Radomsky, Dana Thordarson, and Maureen Whittal.

Contents

INTRODUCTION

The valuable progress made in treating compulsive behaviour, notably compulsive cleaning and compulsive checking, was not accompanied by comparable progress in dealing with obsessions. In recognition of this fact, most researchers conducting therapeutic outcome trials on obsessive-compulsive disorder (OCD) excluded patients whose primary problem was obsessions, estimated to be as many as every third patient. The exclusionary criteria filtered out 'patients with pure obsessions', because behaviour therapists were equipped to deal with observable behaviour but not with inaccessible cognitions.

Finally, progress has been made and obsessions are now more amenable to treatment. This manual describes a focused, specific treatment for obsessions. In order to assist therapists to deal with obsessions this manual provides information, tactics, and techniques that are derived from our new understanding of obsessions and the results of exploratory clinical research. Outcome trials are planned and some are in progress.

The treatment described in this manual is designed for use with patients whose primary or sole problem is obsessions, with or without accompanying compulsions. Between 20 and 30% of the patients who are diagnosed as suffering from an OCD complain that their major or sole problem is obsessions (Stein *et al.* 1997). A recent US national screening survey of anxiety problems showed that 'nearly one third of the sample (of people with OCD symptoms) report cognitive symptoms in the absence of behavioural symptoms, such as cleaning or washing' (Welkowitz *et al.* 2000). In the past these patients received the prevailing treatment for OCD and it was hoped that the obsessions would decline spontaneously even though no specific treatment was provided for the obsessions. The prevailing treatments were behaviour therapy (Rachman and Hodgson 1980; Marks 1987) and more recently cognitive behaviour therapy (Craske 1999; McLean and Woody 2001; Steketee 1994; Salkovskis 1985, 1999). Even in the early uses of behaviour therapy it was recognized that obsessions present special difficulties for behaviour therapy given that obsessions are essentially cognitive in nature. In 1983, it was observed that 'the main obstacle to the successful treatment of obsessions is the absence of effective techniques' (Rachman 1983). Little has changed and as recently as 2000, van Oppen and Emmelkamp concluded that, 'Until now, the treatment of pure obsessions can be summarized as difficult and often unsuccessful' (p. 129). There is however, one encouraging indication that obsessions can be successfully treated. Freeston and colleagues (1997) had rewarding results with a combination of cognitive tactics and traditional exposure methods ('exposure and response prevention is the core of the treatment package', p. 406). Two-thirds of their 29 patients showed clinically significant changes. More needs to be done, and a fully cognitive approach, derived from a firm theory, is expected to help a larger percentage of patients, and hopefully, do so more economically. The Freeston treatment consisted of one and a half hour sessions, up to 40 in total. The average was 25.7 sessions. The core of the present treatment is cognitive, with the emphasis on modifying the patient's catastrophic interpretations of their intrusive thoughts.

It is reasonable to expect that a cognitive problem such as obsessions is best tackled by cognitive means. Hence, the techniques set out in this manual are essentially cognitive, and even more important, the plan and goal of the treatment is to engineer the critical changes in interpretation. The tactics are specific to obsessions, unlike the prevailing methods of treatment. Moreover, they are derived from a theory developed specifically to explain obsessions. The theory and the treatment are new and specific. At present there is no other specific theory to account for obsessions.

For patients who suffer from other types of OCD problems, such as cleaning or checking compulsions, the prevailing cognitive behaviour therapy (CBT) methods are most appropriate. If however, the patients complain in addition that they suffer from obsessions, the techniques described in this manual can be used to supplement the standard OCD treatments as described by Foa and Wilson, Steketee, Salkovskis, and others (see reviews by Abramowitz 1997; Foa *et al.* 1998a; Craske 1999).

How to use this manual: the manual attempts to provide an orderly, practical, and full treatment protocol but because of the subtle and idiosyncratic nature of obsessions, flexibility is essential. The assessment section (Chapter 3) and Stages 1 and 2 of the treatment (Chapters 4 and 5) are essential. Chapter 6 consists of tactics for coping with self-defeating safety behaviour and the specific tactics should be selected as appropriate for the particular case. Chapter 7 describes techniques and tactics for dealing with the different forms of obsessions and can be used as required for the particular case.

Randomized controlled evaluations of psychological therapy are the required standard in psychology and psychiatry, but before one can carry out such trials it is essential to have a clearly described, reproducible, treatment protocol, indeed a treatment manual. This manual provides a protocol for the controlled evaluation of the specific, cognitive treatment of obsessions.

Obsessions and OCD

Obsessions (recurrent, intrusive, unwanted, repugnant thoughts) are a symptom of OCD (Rachman and Hodgson, 1980; Rachman and Shafran, 1998). Repetitive, stereotypic, purposeful, driven compulsive behaviour is the other major symptom of OCD. The most common compulsions are excessive cleaning and/or checking (see Rachman 2001, 2002). In most cases the affected person will experience obsessions and compulsions, with one or other symptom predominating. However, in a significant minority of instances the person suffers primarily from obsessions or from compulsions—the symptoms of obsessions and of compulsions are sufficient to reach a diagnosis of OCD but not necessary.

Compulsions are observable actions and are therefore more amenable to techniques that are designed to modify behaviour. The single most successful technique for overcoming compulsive behaviour is exposure plus response prevention (Rachman and Hodgson 1980; Foa and Wilson 1991; Steketee 1994). This technique can also be helpful in easing the patient's obsessions but it usually does so in an indirect way. Exposure and response prevention is not, and was not, designed to treat internal, cognitive activity such as obsessions. The treatment described in this manual is designed specifically to deal with obsessions.

For patients who are burdened with compulsions as well as obsessions, the addition of standard exposure and response prevention exercises is required (see Steketee 1994). In cases in which the obsessions predominate, the main thrust of treatment should follow the cognitive techniques in this manual. In cases in which the compulsions predominate, the main thrust of treatment should be exposure plus response prevention, supplemented when necessary by these cognitive tactics for dealing with the obsessions.

Preparing a manual for the treatment of obsessions presents special problems because the phenomenon is so subtle, complex, and idiosyncratic as to elude standardization. This accentuates the unavoidable conflict in all manuals between unvaryingly regular procedures and the need to preserve flexibility. The contents of obsessions are limited in range but the personal significance that the sufferer attaches to the occurrence of their obsession can vary widely. Hence the approach to the general content and nature of the obsessions is reasonably standardized, but in dealing with the personal significance of the obsessions, flexible guidelines are set out.

This manual combines cognitive and behavioural components. The cognitive components are derived from the cognitive theory that unwanted, intrusive thoughts (images or impulses) turn into obsessions if the affected person interprets these thoughts as having important personal significance. The thoughts are interpreted by the person as being revealing, and as signifying that he/she is immoral, evil, dangerous, insane, or has a combination of these qualities. They may believe that the thoughts will lead to catastrophic consequences, and tend to fear that they will lose control. Hence, the thoughts are distressing and give rise to attempts to put matters right, to neutralize, to conceal, or to suppress the thoughts, and to avoid anxiety-provoking places or people.

The primary aim of the treatment is to assist the patient to make more realistic and accurate interpretations of the significance of their unwanted, intrusive thoughts. This involves an analysis of the thoughts and the meaning and interpretations the patient places on them, the therapeutic collection of evidence (especially in behavioural experiments), reasons for and against the interpretations, the generation of alternative interpretations and their evaluation, attempts to eliminate thought suppression, neutralization and avoidance behaviour. The treatment program has a large and important educational component, and involves the collection and evaluation of data at each stage.

The emphasis of the treatment is to understand the person's interpretations of his/her intrusive, unwanted thoughts—and then to help modify these interpretations into adaptive and realistic alternatives. The cognitive work is primary but is supplemented by exposure exercises, behavioural experiments, and encouragement to cease avoidance, concealment, thought suppression, internal debates, and neutralization.

Most patients find this course of treatment acceptable and they tend to pass through stages. At the start they are open-minded unless they have already failed to benefit from other treatments, in which case they express a healthy scepticism. As they begin to reveal the content of their obsessions, they can get troubled and even find it to be a painful process. The core cognitive work is mentally taxing and exhausting. When they make solid progress their enthusiasm rises and they carry out a mental house-cleaning. In the best of outcomes they finally experience a sense of liberation.

In order to facilitate and guide the content and sequence of sessions, a Session-by-session progress chart is provided in the Toolkit (form 6), at the end of the manual. It provides a structure for each session and is used in a flexible way to accommodate the particular problems of each patient. The Toolkit contains copies of specially devised forms and charts that will enable the therapist to structure the treatment and provide direction and tactics. Therapists are free to reproduce as many copies as they require (except for tests that are covered by other authors'/publishers' rights, as indicated in the text).

CHAPTER 1

The nature of obsessions

Obsessions are repetitive, unwanted thoughts, images, or impulses that a person finds unacceptable and/or repugnant. They are among the most distressing psychological problems and can be mentally exhausting. Struggling against obsessions is a lonely, private battle. The three main themes of obsessions are unacceptable aggressive, sexual, or blasphemous thoughts. The person is distressed by these unwanted, repugnant, and seemingly inexplicable impulses, images, or thoughts. Obsessions generally give rise to resistance, fighting off the thought, attempting to neutralize the effect of the thought, to cancel it, or to put matters right. They can also give rise to extensive avoidance behaviour. In recent years, the term 'obsessional' has been broadened, in some circumstances, to mean more than a classical obsession: it is applied to include all thoughts associated with compulsive behaviour. This manual deals with classical obsessions, the repugnant and unacceptable intrusive thoughts that conflict with the person's self-view and are resisted.

The term 'obsessions' is sometimes used to encompass recurrent, preoccupying thoughts. In the DSM system of classification, for example, 'obsessions' include recurrent, preoccupying thoughts about checking, washing, and similar compulsive behaviour, but these thoughts lack the repugnant, often violent, immoral, objectionable qualities of classical obsessions and seldom give rise to resistance. The objectionable, immoral intrusive thoughts, classical obsessions, invariably give rise to resistance. The broader use of the term emphasizes recurrence and preoccupation, but does not require the elements of repugnance and resistance.

Examples of classical obsessions include the following.

1 Aggressive (or harm) obsessions, such as thoughts of harming old people or children or relatives (I will push an elderly man under the oncoming train; I will stab my mother; I will throw rocks at children) or thoughts of harm coming to relatives/friends (my parents will be brutally assaulted by an intruder). Many of these harm obsessions involve violence.

2 Sexual obsessions include: fear of inappropriate acts or gestures (I will sexually molest a young child; I will expose myself in a public place), and repeated images of sex with inappropriate partners (I see myself having sex

with a religious figure; I experience sexual thoughts about my sister/brother, mother/father). Sexual obsessions are more common among men than women.

3 Blasphemous obsessions include: a fear of making sacrilegious gestures in a holy place (I will shout foul, obscene language in church), the pollution of prayers or other rituals by impure, disgusting thoughts (the intrusion of foul language during prayers).

Some obsessions combine elements of two or more of these three major themes: sex, aggression, blasphemy. One patient who was assailed by bizarre, repugnant, violent images and thoughts described it as living in a nightmare, 'only I am awake'.

People experiencing obsessions recognize that the thoughts are their own production, and find them to be ego-dystonic (contrary to their view of themselves). As a result of these features, combined with the objectionable quality of the content of the obsessions, the person generally resists the obsessions. The affected person tries to block the intrusive ideas, to oppose them, suppress them, debate them, or reject them altogether. The obsessions can produce feelings of shame, disgust, fear, self-doubt, and self-distrust. People tend to question their view of themselves and their morality, and may begin to feel that they are unsafe, evil, weird, or on the verge of going crazy. The thoughts are so shameful/embarrassing that people prefer to conceal them, and feel guilty for having such unacceptable and repugnant ideas.

The major misinterpretations can be summarized in this way: these horrible thoughts mean that I am bad, mad, or dangerous—or all three.

Most obsessions are kept secret—in one patient's words, 'It is my dirty little secret'. Another patient said, after successful treatment, that 'the number of my secrets was a measure of my illness'. Before entering therapy, they tend to believe that their obsessional experiences are unique to them, and this belief is protected by keeping the experiences secret. It follows that they feel they are freakish and/or weird. Given that most of the people who are seriously affected by obsessions have high moral and/or religious standards, these ideas are extremely objectionable and give rise to self-doubt, self-distrust, feelings of degradation, and anxiety about their true personality. They fear that the obsessional experiences indicate that they have lurking inside their seemingly virtuous personality, secret thoughts and ideas that are dangerous, wicked, disturbing, sinful, and unsafe (e.g. 'I must be a very bad person?'). Many patients are intensely fearful that one day they will lose control and carry out the repugnant actions. As will be described presently, it can be didactic to help the patient calculate the number of times that they have had the thoughts or impulses (usually thousands and thousands of times) and the total absence of consequent actions. For example, a 30-year-old woman was deeply troubled by her recurrent thoughts of aggression towards others. Given that she had such thoughts every single day, repeatedly, over a period of 12 years, we concluded from our rough calculation that she had racked up a score of some 300 000 aggressive obsessional thoughts. On the other side of the balance, she could not recall carrying out a single aggressive action throughout the 12-year period of her struggle with obsessive compulsive disorder (OCD).

In some cases of OCD, people suffer from a feeling of mental pollution (Rachman 1994) in addition to their other concerns. This feeling of an internal, immoral dirtiness, can also enter into classical obsessions. People who are assailed by repugnant and distressing thoughts or images of bizarre/unacceptable sexual acts can feel polluted, as can people who are besieged by vile and blasphemous thoughts. Feelings of mental/moral pollution give rise to excessive cleaning and purification, but the cleaning rarely achieves peace.

The three forms of obsessions—thoughts, images, impulses—have many features in common (intrusiveness, unacceptability, and so on), but differences between them can be of therapeutic significance. In factor analytical studies, distress and uncontrollability emerged as the main factors of all obsessions (Rachman and Hodgson 1980). On a number of measures, however, obsessional impulses were rated as the most unpleasant of the three. They were reported to be more intense, more distressing, more tormenting, and more difficult to deal with than the images or thoughts. Clinically, they more often lead to avoidance behaviour; for example, patients who experience obsessional impulses to harm children tend to avoid public play areas, schools, and so on. Obsessional images tend to be of shorter duration and are more easily dismissed or broken by distraction. Obsessional thoughts are the most common form, and sometimes dwell on past events, such as guilty ruminations about past actions or failures to act.

It appears that anxiety does most to promote frequent intrusions, and dysphoria does most to prolong the intrusions. To a surprising extent, obsessions are triggered by external precipitants, a finding that is taken into account by incorporating exposure exercises in treatment programmes. As the connection between external cues and 'internal intrusive cognitions' is not always obvious, the value of exposure exercises tends to be overlooked. It is probable that repeated exercises reduce the patient's anxiety and lead to important cognitive changes, such as, 'I did not attack any children, I am not a dangerous person'.

Given the role of anxiety and dysphoria in provoking and maintaining obsessional intrusions, some benefits can be achieved by dealing with the aversive effects by indirect means, that is, by treating the dysphoria/anxiety.

Table 1.1 Forms of obsessions

	Thoughts	Images	Impulses
Intrusive	Yes	Yes	Yes
Unwanted	Yes	Yes	Yes
Repugnant	Yes	Yes	Yes
Objectionable	Yes	Yes	Yes
Resisted	Yes	Yes	Yes
Pictures in the mind	No	Yes	No
Frightening	Yes	Yes	Extremely
Fear of loss of control	Yes	Yes	Intense
Avoidance	Yes	Yes	Intense
Immorality	Yes	Intense	Yes
Neutralizing attempts	Yes	Intense	Yes
Agitation	Yes	Yes	Intense
Frustration	Extreme	Extreme	Yes
Duration	Often prolonged	Fleeting	Can be brief

Examples:

Images of incestuous acts, images of blinding a child.

Thoughts of serious harm coming to parents, blasphemous thoughts about the Virgin Mary.

Impulses to push an elderly person in the path of an oncoming train, impulses to expose oneself in public, impulses to sexually molest a young child.

The person's ability to dismiss their obsessions is related to the intensity and the distressing power of the intrusions, and the distress produced by the obsessions is influenced by the person's affective state. It follows that success in improving the patient's affective state should reduce the distress caused by the obsessions and, hence, make it easier to dismiss them. The value of the indirect tactics of reducing dysphoria/anxiety, by psychological or pharmacological means, is understandable, and they are compatible with the direct tactics that form the substance of the manual.

Avoidance behaviour

Even though obsessions are essentially cognitive, the behavioural component can be very important and should not be neglected. People who are tormented by obsessional impulses to make violent attacks take great care to avoid sharp instruments, weapons, potential victims, and so on. Those who have obsessional thoughts of deliberately causing a motor vehicle accident, avoid driving. As in other forms of cognitive behaviour therapy, the patient is encouraged to reduce the maladaptive avoidance behaviour. If the patient experiences excessive anxiety, relaxation exercises may facilitate the early exposure exercises and can also be used during the exposure session, as needed. Whenever appropriate, the therapist begins by providing therapeutic modelling sessions. These sessions help to reduce the patient's fear and avoidance, and also serve to restore the person's belief in his/her dependability. They have to regain the belief in themselves as safe people. Numerous obsessions are provoked by external cues, such as sharp objects, and they can provide the material for successful exposure exercises, as in straightforward behaviour therapy. Patients who experience obsessional impulses of violence tend to avoid horror movies, sharp knives, and kitchens—because they have learnt that these stimuli can trigger their obsessional impulses. Patients experiencing objectionable sexual images avoid explicitly sexual movies, magazines, and pictures, for fear of triggering their obsessions. An unfortunate consequence of avoidance is that the person reduces the chances of gaining disconfirming evidence; the maladaptive cognitions are preserved.

During the assessment phase it is important to collect information about avoidance behaviour and, whenever possible, conduct a set of behavioural avoidance tests.

Responsibility for thoughts

Some people with OCD hold extreme beliefs about beliefs; for example, they may believe that they should be able fully to control their thoughts. In particular, they feel that they must control their objectionable, supposedly important, and revealing thoughts.

Patients are surprised and often relieved to learn that all people experience intrusive thoughts, many of them unwanted thoughts. They are relieved of some guilt and also are relieved to learn that their intrusive experiences are not a sign of mental illness; they learn that their experiences and thoughts need not be concealed or feared. The intrusive, unwanted thoughts do not lead to disaster. They are a psychological phenomenon in their own right, are commonly experienced, and not a way-station to losing control or to insanity.

Affected people tend to attach undue significance to their intrusive thoughts, and this over-interpretation can become entangled with their exaggerated sense of responsibility (Rachman 1997c; Salkovskis 1985, 1999; Purdon 1999). For example, 'My immoral sexual thoughts reveal something important and unflattering about the kind of person that I really am', and this can be entangled with 'I am morally responsible for these objectionable thoughts'. It can even extend to the psychological fusion of the thought and action (see below). People who regard their homosexual thoughts as unacceptable, sometimes reason in this way: 'My intrusive thoughts about homosexuality are unacceptable and indicate that I am fundamentally homosexual in preference'. A comparable chain of reasoning can occur with blasphemous thoughts. People feel that the mere experience of having a blasphemous thought is equivalent to committing an act of blasphemy, and consequently they are sinfully responsible.

The majority of people dismiss or ignore their unwanted intrusive thoughts and regard them as dross. However, once a person attaches important meaning to these unwanted thoughts, they tend to become distressing and adhesive. The full causes of the process by which obsessions acquire extraordinary significance for a person are not always evident. The inclination to over-interpret the significance of our intrusive thoughts is perhaps promoted by direct instruction, moral or religious. Strict moral education may also promote elevated levels of personal responsibility. The tendency to over-interpret can also arise from direct experiences or as a result of self-instruction.

Elevated responsibility leads to attempts to protect other people. Obsessions involving harm lead to attempts to prevent other people from the harm signalled by the obsession. This can be attempted by carrying out a neutralizing action or by forming a neutralizing thought or counter-image or counter-thought.

Hostility

During the course of treatment it is not uncommon to observe signs of hostility, particularly among patients who are disturbed by their recurrent thoughts/impulses to harm other people. The patients are troubled and distressed by the frequency and nastiness of these aggressive thoughts, as they almost invariably have high standards of personal conduct. They try to be considerate and go to lengths to avoid upsetting others, let alone causing them serious harm. As one patient put it, 'I seem to be a confusion of Mother Theresa and a serial killer'.

Numbers of clinicians are of the opinion, possibly correct, that obsessional patients have difficulty in expressing their anger. The notion that the patients' expressions of great concern for others, and their excessively kind and considerate actions, are over-compensations, reaction formations, to their unacceptable feelings of anger has its origin in psychoanalytic thinking. The difficulties in conducting adequate research in psychoanalysis led to the neglect of the idea, but within the past few years conventional, psychometric, research has produced some evidence of elevated hostility/anger among patients with anxiety disorders. For example, Dadds *et al.* (1993), found that intropunitive hostility was a feature of these disorders. Comparable findings were reported by Rocca *et al.* (1998): their 30 patients with OCD reported the highest scores on hostility but discordantly low scores on the expression of anger. Similarly, we found that among 160 non-clinical students, hostility was the best predictor of high scores on an OCD scale (S. Rachman 1999, unpublished). However, the high scorers on the OCD scale had low to average scores on the expression of anger. The results are consistent with the possibility that patients with harm obsessions do have elevated feelings of hostility but suppress their expression. The connection between hostility and harm obsessions was clearly evident in a patient receiving cognitive behaviour therapy. He made gratifyingly satisfactory progress in reinterpreting his intrusive thoughts and their frequency declined; however, when he had upsetting encounters or conversations with people whom he felt were critical of him, the frequency of the harm obsessions spiked up briefly. Harm obsessions can also be provoked by exposure to aggressive movies or other material, in keeping with the important research reported by Horowitz (1975). In a number of experiments he demonstrated that the frequency and aversiveness of intrusive thoughts is increased by exposure to stressful material.

In many instances their hostility is understandably reactive to ill-treatment by family, friends, and so on, but when the ensuing feelings of hostility come into conflict with the value they attach to considerate and kind behaviour, they try to suppress the expression of their anger. The recurrent intrusive and angry thoughts are unacceptable and are therefore resisted, but without success. One aspect of this difficulty may arise from an exaggerated sense of responsibility, and the tendency therefore to assign the blame internally rather than externally. On those occasions when they do assign blame elsewhere, their anger is in no doubt. Following this analysis through, the clinical dictum that obsessional patients sometimes make progress when they learn to express anger, can be interpreted as a redirection of their excessive responsibility and of their excessively internal attributions.

If responsibility for an anticipated or actual misfortune is redirected away from oneself toward another person or agency, anger may follow. Therapists should be prepared for patients to experience some anger in place of their pervasive guilt, if and when a re-attribution of responsibility occurs. In these instances, the therapist should help to explain the nature and cause of the new anger and assist the patient to acquire a balanced view of the allocation of responsibility, and also of behaviour that is appropriate and effective when feelings of anger arise.

Thought–action fusion

Thought–action fusion (TAF) is a phenomenon in which people tend to regard their thoughts as being psychologically equivalent to the corresponding action, and/or to believe that their thoughts of possible misfortunes actually increase the likelihood that the misfortune will occur. It is almost as wicked to think of pushing an elderly man on to a railway track as it would be to actually push him. Additionally, the thought of pushing an elderly man on to a railway track is believed to actually increase the risk to that person. The unwanted intrusive image of having sex with a religious figure is an immoral equivalent of carrying out the act itself. Two forms of TAF have been identified: perceived probability TAF, in which the intrusive thought increases the probability of the unacceptable event occurring; and moral TAF, in which the thought is shameful and morally equivalent to the event (see Rachman and Shafran 1998). Probability TAF feeds into fears of losing control, and moral TAF is strongly associated with feelings of guilt and responsibility.

A cognitive theory of obsession

This treatment is based on the cognitive theory that obsessions are caused by catastrophic misinterpretations of the significance of one's unwanted intrusive thoughts, images, impulses (Rachman 1997c, 1998). By deduction: (a) the obsessions will persist for as long as the misinterpretations continue; and (b) the obsessions will diminish or disappear as a function of the weakening/ elimination of the misinterpretations.

The unacknowledged assumption that obsessions are categorically separable, that obsessions are pathological and qualitatively different from other intrusive thoughts, was a barrier to progress. The obstacle was removed by conceptualizing obsessions as unwanted and unacceptable intrusive thoughts, and by the demonstration that such obsessional experiences are nigh universal (Rachman 1971, 1976a; Rachman and de Silva 1978; Salkovskis and Harrison 1984). An essentially cognitive disorder, such as obsession, requires an essentially cognitive explanation.

The behavioural approach focused on disorders of (observable) behaviour and was therefore equipped to tackle compulsive repetitive behaviour such as compulsive cleaning and checking. It was unable to tackle the unobservable and inaccessible obsessions—hence the routine exclusion of patients with 'pure obsessions' from behavioural research and treatment trials.

A cognitive understanding of obsession

This theory is an explicit attempt to expand Clark's (1986) theory of panic to obsessions, and draws heavily from Salkovskis's profoundly important (1985) cognitive analysis of OCD (see also de Silva 1994; Freeston *et al.* 1996; Salkovskis and Kirk 1997). The theory is constructed on the work of Clark and Salkovskis.

The core statement regarding misinterpretations of one's intrusive thoughts is deliberately succinct and simple. The theory and deductions are testable, encompass a range of observations and findings, draw strength from experimental and clinical research on panic, and, if confirmed, will justify the practical implementation of focused therapy for obsessions. The starting point for the theory is the premise that unwanted, intrusive thoughts are the raw material of obsessions, and the finding that these thoughts are almost universally experienced.

Obsessions are defined as 'intrusive, repetitive thoughts, images or impulses that are unacceptable and/or unwanted and give rise to subjective resistance . . . the necessary and sufficient conditions . . . are intrusiveness, internal attribution, unwantedness and difficulty of control' (Rachman and Hodgson 1980, p. 251). Obsessional intrusive thoughts are similar in some ways to the unwanted intrusive thoughts (images or impulses) that nearly everyone experiences, but there are also some differences: they are more intense, longer lasting, more insistent, more distressing, and more adhesive than the common variety of intrusive thoughts (Rachman and de Silva 1978). However, the form and content of abnormal and normal intrusive thoughts are similar. The characteristics of compulsions, morbid preoccupations, contamination fears, and related, but different, OCD phenomena, are described in Rachman and Hodgson (1980). The present theory is a theory of obsessions. Compulsions are repetitive, intense, stereotypic actions, such as cleaning or checking, that the person carries out in order to remove a perceived threat (e.g. of being contaminated) or to prevent a future threat (e.g. of causing a fire). The affected person feels compelled to carry out the actions, but can prolong, extend, curtail, or delay the actions.

What causes the transition from a normal intrusive thought into an abnormal obsession? Given the nature and distinguishing characteristics of the abnormal intrusive thoughts, plus Salkovskis's (1985) astute and critical emphasis on the meaning of the thought for the person, it is plausible that a catastrophic misinterpretation of the significance of the thought produces the very qualities that are distinctive of the abnormal obsessions. The misinterpretation of the intrusive thoughts as being very important, personally significant, revealing, and threatening or even catastrophic, has the effect of transforming a commonplace nuisance into a torment. The catastrophic misinterpretations often give rise to additional fears of the possible consequences of the obsessions: 'Will it lead me to attack someone?', 'Will the obsessions drive me insane?', and so on.

These are some case examples of catastrophic misinterpretations of obsessions. A 25-year-old computer analyst had recurrent thoughts and images of harming the very young children of a close friend, and interpreted this to mean that he is potential murderer, and a fundamentally evil and worthless human being. A second patient, devoutly religious, had recurrent and violent obscene images about the church and Mary, especially in church or when she tried to pray. She interpreted them to mean that she was a vicious, lying hypocrite, and that her religious beliefs and feelings were a sham. An affectionate and attentive grandmother had recurrent images of throwing her beloved grandson over the balcony and the resultant distress brought her close to suicide; she interpreted the images to mean that she was a dangerous and uncontrollable psychopath, and a person incapable of love or concern for other people. After a successful course of cognitive behaviour therapy (CBT) the obsessions were wiped out and she was able to resume a normal life, fully enjoying her grandchild.

Several arguments and lines of evidence can be assembled in support of the theory (see Rachman 1997c, 1998). They are based on the following findings: cognitions can cause anxiety, anxiety provoking interpretations of cognitions can lead to obsessions, and particular cognitive biases are associated with vulnerability to obsessions.

Cognitions can cause anxiety

First, the important functional connection between cognitions and anxiety has been demonstrated in research and treatment studies of the cognitive theory of panic (see: Clark 1986, 1988, 1996, 1997; Ehlers 1993; McNally 1994). People with panic disorder are more likely to make catastrophic misinterpretations of bodily sensations than are other people. The theory of obsession assumes that there is an essential similarity between obsession and panic. Both theories attribute the disorder to catastrophic misinterpretations of thoughts/sensations, and share many features. However, panic is episodic and obsession tends towards constancy. The intrusive thoughts that provide the raw material for obsession tend towards a daily constancy, and patients complain that the nasty thoughts are always present, even when they are merely lurking 'at the back of my mind'. There is a sense that they are always hovering.

Catastrophic interpretations lead to obsession

Secondly, patients afflicted by recurrent obsessions commonly attach exaggerated significance to these thoughts and regard them as horrific, repugnant, threatening, dangerous, or all of these (e.g. see Freeston *et al.* 1993). Various patients have described their obsessional thoughts, impulses, or images as: immoral, sinful, disgusting, revealing, dangerous, threatening, alarming, predictive, insane, bewildering, and criminal. At a higher level, they interpreted these thoughts, impulses, or images as revealing important but usually hidden elements in their character, such as: these obsessions mean that deep down I am an evil person; I am dangerous; I am unreliable; I may become totally uncontrollable (see especially Purdon and Clark 1994); I am weird; I am going insane (and will lose control?); I am a sinful person; I am fundamentally immoral. Some of the elaborations of the interpretations lead them to fear specific consequences, such as: one day I will lose control (and perhaps act upon my violent, aggressive, immoral impulses?); one day I will break down and cause serious physical harm to others; if other people knew about my obsessions and/or their content, they would completely reject me; one day I will be locked up; I will be sent to hell; I am being (will be, deserve to be) punished.

The main themes of obsessions—aggression, sex, and blasphemy—are important themes of all moral systems, and hence open to an inflation of personal significance. (Incidentally, it is interesting that people rarely have obsessions about strong people who are well capable of defending themselves; it is usually children, disabled, or elderly people who feature because unwanted thoughts about harming helpless people are interpreted as being particularly shocking and reprehensible.)

It is evident from this analysis that in the cognitive theory of obsession, the *content* of the obsessions is of critical concern. Elsewhere it has been observed that cognitive theory, in general, is providing content to the behavioural theories (Rachman 1997a).

Given these descriptions, interpretations, and anticipated consequences, it is no surprise that the obsessions are so repugnant and frightening to the affected person, and their intense even frantic attempts to resist or remove the obsessions are perfectly understandable. So too is the avoidance behaviour that is generated by the obsessions. For example, a recurrent image of stabbing her children led a patient vigorously to avoid any contact with sharp objects and she had strong locks installed on the kitchen doors. She was unable to enter or remain in her kitchen unless accompanied by a trusted adult.

Attempts to neutralize are attempts to prevent or mitigate the anticipated effects of the obsession. The person has a strong urge to cancel, correct, counteract, or atone for the obsession—in the familiar phrase, to 'put matters right'. Attempts at neutralization can be frustrating and exhausting. Patients describe this sense of exhaustion even after spending a seemingly quiet and inactive day at home. Relatives are often puzzled and even irritated by these complaints, 'But you have done nothing all day!'. As with compulsions, to which acts of neutralization bear a strong resemblance, the urge to act is strengthened by the fact that compulsions and neutralizations are partly successful; they relieve some part of the discomfort the person experiences from the obsessions (Rachman and Hodgson 1980; Rachman *et al.* 1996). However, it now appears possible that the relief accomplished by neutralization would have occurred spontaneously (Rachman *et al.* 1996). After an inactive delay period, the discomfort declines as it does after neutralization; the urge to neutralize also declines spontaneously, but more slowly (see Chapter 2). Presumably neutralization persists because it succeeds, but as with compulsions, this temporary relief comes at a price. Indirectly the neutralization helps to preserve the causal misinterpretations and their anticipated consequences.

Cognitive biases in obsessions

There is ample evidence of the operation of cognitive biases in our thinking (Tversky and Kahneman 1974; Nisbett and Ross 1980), and more recently in the operation of cognitive biases in OCD. For example, Lopatka and Rachman (1995) found that people with obsessional problems tend to think that the probability of a disaster or unpleasant event is increased when they are responsible. They are also inclined to think that they, but not other people, can be held responsible for misfortunes over which they have no control whatsoever. Additionally, there is a relationship between OCD and a cognitive bias of TAF (Rachman 1993; Shafran *et al.* 1996; see Chapter 2).

Insofar as a person uses (or is subject to?) cognitive biases, the vulnerability to abnormal obsessions is increased. Ultimately, we will need to explain, in addition, the origin and persistence of these biases, but that is a difficult task because the origin of even the common biases, such as the representativeness bias, remains to be fully explained. There appears to be a connection between an inflated sense of responsibility, as described by Salkovskis (1985), and the operation of specific OCD biases such as TAF (Rachman 1993). We have experimental evidence that an increased sense of responsibility for an unwanted event can lead to an increased estimate of the probability that the unwanted event will occur (Lopatka and Rachman 1995; Rachman 1997c). 'If I am responsible for ensuring the safety of the house, the probability of a fire occurring is significantly greater than it would be if you were responsible for its safety', or more broadly, 'When I am responsible, things are more likely to go wrong'. Given that the estimated probability of an aversive event and the estimated seriousness of the consequences are important contributors to anxiety (e.g. see Butler and Mathews 1987; van Oppen and Arntz 1994; Freeston *et al.* 1996; Rachman 1997b), this particular bias is a likely contributor to anxiety.

The related bias, a feeling of responsibility even in the absence of control can be illustrated by a patient who felt responsible for ensuring the day-to-day safety of his parents who lived in a town 200 miles away. He attempted to protect them (actually to reduce his distress) by repeated hand washing.

These biases have been demonstrated in patients (Lopatka and Rachman 1995) and in students (Shafran *et al.* 1996). In a group of 214 students, significant correlations were found between these two biases and scores on the Maudsley Obsessional Compulsive Inventory (Hodgson and Rachman 1977), and also between these biases and the TAF bias. Moreover, the 28 subjects with a high total bias score reported significantly more obsessions (and other OCD-type features) than did the 38 subjects with a low total bias score.

The lack of success of pre-cognitive theory and treatments for obsessions

Treatment techniques were deduced from the earlier, behavioural analysis of OCD, and the analysis was also used to accommodate *ad hoc* procedures, such as thought-stopping. With few exceptions these special procedures were unsuccessful.

The unsuccessful tactics were thought-stopping, a rubber band sting on the wrist, and habituation training (Stern *et al.* 1973; Parkinson and Rachman 1980; Likierman and Rachman 1982; Marks 1987). It now appears that these techniques were unsuccessful because they arose from, or were justified by, an unsatisfactory theory of obsession. Moreover, in the light of the cognitive theory of obsession, these failures can be post-dicted. The techniques were attempts to block or reduce the manifestations of the problem, but neglected the underlying problem, that is the catastrophic misinterpretations of the significance of the intrusive thoughts were left unchanged.

So, even if the tactic of thought-stopping is applied rigorously, which is difficult, the most that can be expected is a temporary abortion or suppression of the obsessions (incidentally, there is some, not wholly consistent, evidence that active suppression can cause a temporary increase in the intrusive thoughts; Salkovskis 1996). For similar reasons, the administration of a sting by a rubber band strapped to the wrist, which is a form of thought-interruption, also has a limited, temporary effect, if any.

Habituation training (also called satiation) was deduced directly from a behavioural 'anatomy of obsessions' (Rachman 1978). It was argued that, just as habituation training is capable of reducing fears, for a period at least, construing the obsessions as fear/discomfort-producing events, the repeated evocation of the obsession should reduce the associated discomfort. The results of an experimental investigation of 12 patients showed that habituation training, and separately thought-stopping, produced small changes at best, and these soon faded (Likierman and Rachman 1982). It is probable that these attempts failed because they did nothing to change the distressing misinterpretations of the intrusive thoughts and merely damped down the effects of the misinterpretations. As the misinterpretations presumably persisted, the distressing obsessions soon reappeared.

Where do the obsessions come from?

A complete answer to this question must wait for the time, not imminent, when we have a better grasp on the very nature of human thinking. At this stage, however, two facts about the origins of obsessions are worth remarking. First, we know that exposure to stress increases the incidence of unwanted intrusive thoughts, which are, after all, the raw material for full obsessions. Secondly, a surprisingly large number of obsessional thoughts (and especially impulses) are triggered by external cues (Rachman and de Silva 1978). The belief that obsessions are essentially, exclusively, internally generated has not been confirmed.

Fuller accounts of these two observations are given in Rachman (1978), Rachman and de Silva (1978) and Rachman and Hodgson (1980) but the essence of each is as follows. Patients report that during stress, their obsessions increase in frequency. The experimental research of Horowitz (1975), in which patients (and non-patients) reported increases in intrusive thoughts when exposed to stressful material, such as films, is consistent with this. In a naturalistic study, Parkinson and Rachman (1980) found that the mothers of children awaiting surgery experienced steep increases in unwanted intrusive thoughts—and a rapid decline when the child was safely out of surgery. Obsessions also increase during periods of dysphoria (Rachman and de Silva 1978) and Ricciardi and McNally (1995) have neatly confirmed the long-standing belief in a close connection between depression and obsessions: in a case-series analysis of 150 patients, they found that 'mood disorders seem selectively associated with a worsening of obsessions' (p. 249). It remains to be determined whether dysphoria provides fertile soil for the intrusive thoughts, or whether it also provokes them. Either way, the present theory needs to be developed to include this connection—perhaps in a state of dysphoria, the significance and/or feared consequences of the intrusive thoughts are given a nasty twist?

The second observation, of the surprisingly large impact of external cues, was originally encountered in a study of the similarities and differences between normal and abnormal obsessions, and, as mentioned above, external provocation (and hence, more intense avoidance perhaps?) was especially important in stirring obsessive impulses. The research by Horowitz (1975) provides broad confirmation of the provocation of intrusive thoughts by external stressors (see Rachman and Hodgson 1980 for a summary account).

As in panic, it is likely that unfortunate sufferers from obsessions get caught up in a vicious circle.

Why do they persist?

The obsessions persist for as long as the misinterpretations persist, and these in turn will continue unless and until new evidence and/or arguments overturn the misinterpretations.

Why are the obsessions so frequent? Probably because the person's catastrophic misinterpretations of the intrusive thoughts result in a conversion of neutral cues and contexts into dangerous cues and contexts (Rachman 1998).

The relationship between significant misinterpretations and the frequency of obsessions

It remains to be explained how a catastrophic misinterpretation of the significance of an intrusive, unwanted thought causes a paradoxical increase in the frequency of the obsession, and how it also contributes to the remarkable persistence of the obsession. What is the connection between the significance attached to the obsession, and its frequency and persistence?

To begin with, we know that the frequency of intrusive thoughts is increased when people are subjected to stressful material or experiences (Horowitz 1975; Rachman and Hodgson 1980). In brief, the more stressful the material, the greater the number of intrusive thoughts and the greater the distress that they evoke. We also know that an increase in the number of threatening stimuli is also followed by an increase in the number of intrusive thoughts (Horowitz 1975; Parkinson and Rachman 1980).

It is argued here that when a person makes a catastrophic misinterpretation of the significance of his unwanted intrusive thoughts, this will increase the range and seriousness of potentially threatening stimuli. A wide range of stimuli are converted from neutrality into threat. Previously indifferent stimuli become highly salient. So, for example, if a person catastrophically misinterprets his unwanted intrusive thoughts about harming other people as signifying that he is potentially dangerous, then a range of formerly neutral stimuli are turned into potential threats (e.g. sharp objects are transformed into potential weapons).

This conversion of neutral cues and situations into potentially threatening ones increases the range of threats and therefore increases the opportunities for the provocation of obsessions. To continue with the same example, if my catastrophic misinterpretation leads to the conversion of sharp objects from neutral to threatening, then the opportunities for provocation of the unwanted thoughts are greatly increased by the addition of this new and wide range of threats. 'I am dangerous, and hence sharp objects are now viewed as threatening and best avoided.'

The repeated avoidance of sharp objects, unattended children, etc., leaves the person's view of himself as dangerous, unchallenged and unchanged. This same sequence of events can occur with internal stimuli. For example, if the person interprets the intrusive thoughts as signifying that he is dangerous and may lose control and harm a child, it follows that sensations of discomfort/anxiety (e.g. trembling, sweating) in the presence of children are interpreted as impending signs of serious loss of control. There is also a risk here of what Arntz and colleagues (1995) have called ex-consequentia reasoning, in which the person deduces a threat from the fact of feeling anxious. 'If I am anxious, it must mean that there is danger present', and in the present argument, 'If I am anxious when near children, there is a danger present, and I am it!'. Another example is: 'If I am constantly thinking of harming helpless people, it must mean that I am bad and dangerous—I am a significant threat'. Also the anxiety means that I do not have control of my reactions, and therefore there is an increased likelihood that I will act on the unwanted impulse. Hence the catastrophic misinterpretation of one's anxiety can interact to increase the catastrophic misinterpretation of the intrusion.

Anxiety in the presence of children is sometimes misinterpreted by patients as a sign of sexual arousal. 'I feel tense and trembling when I am near this child and it means that I am responding sexually.' This interpretation of internal sensations or external cues as signs of potential threat often leads to avoidance. The person avoids sharp instruments, attending church, being alone with children and, as argued earlier (Rachman 1997c), the avoidance behaviour leaves the catastrophic misinterpretation unchallenged. The opportunities for elicitation of obsessions,

Table 1.2 Analysis of the connection between significance and frequency can be illustrated in a series of steps, with accompanying examples

Step	Significance and frequency of obsessions	Examples
1	Stress increases intrusive thoughts.	
2	Thoughts are given catastrophic significance (danger, loss of control, insanity, evil).	They are very important, and revealing about me. I am dangerous.
Mainly external cues		
3	Given that I am a dangerous person, many situations and cues become salient and are now turned into threats—the range widens.	I am dangerous/evil and may harm others; sharp objects become threat cues.
4	Hence, opportunities for provocation of obsessions increase.	The sight of sharp objects, or unattended children, now provokes obsessions.
5	Avoid threat cues and/or neutralize the thought.	Avoid places where children congregate, avoid knives.
6	The catastrophic significance remains unchanged (or is even confirmed) by the avoidance.	The fact that I cannot be left alone with children proves that I am evil/dangerous.
7	The fact that I am constantly having these thoughts means that there is a danger (why else am I having these thoughts?).	Repeatedly thinking of harming children means that I'm evil/dangerous.
8	Given my dangerousness/wickedness, the range of potentially dangerous cues increases.	It makes me so anxious that I will never agree to care for or ever be alone with an infant —any infant, anywhere, anytime.
9	The opportunities for provocation of obsessions are therefore increased.	Unplanned exposures to infants, sharp objects are not avoidable.
10	This leads to a high frequency of obsessions, particularly in response to the less avoidable, internal cues.	The sight of any infant makes me very anxious and this can provoke harm obsessions.
Mainly internal cues		
11	The increase in the range of threatening cues can take place solely or largely 'internally'—more and more internal cues turn threatening.	I am trembling and sweating in the presence of this infant; I am losing control.
12	The fact that I am anxious in these situations means that I am indeed dangerous (ex-consequentia reasoning).	The intense anxiety caused when I see knives proves that I am untrustworthy/dangerous.

by the widening range of internal sensations or internal stimuli, are increased, and hence, the frequency of the obsessions remains high.

In contrast, if the catastrophic misinterpretation is changed or reduced and replaced by a benign interpretation, the opportunities for the elicitation of the obsessions are reduced. The frequency of the obsessions will decline in large part because of the re-conversion of threat stimuli back to neutral stimuli: there are fewer opportunities for the elicitation of the obsessions.

Which neutral cues are converted into threat stimuli and why? This depends on the specific content of the intrusive thought and its meaning to the affected person. For a deeply religious person, intrusive blasphemous images or thoughts can be interpreted as catastrophic and will cause previously neutral religious cues to become threats (e.g. churches, prayers, religious practices, religious pictures, even religious words). For a person assailed by intrusive thoughts of aggression towards children, any congregation of children becomes a source of threat, being alone with a young child becomes a threat. For a person who begins to experience intrusive thoughts of violence, sharp objects are converted into items of threat. Contrariwise, for the person troubled by blasphemous thoughts, sharp objects remain neutral. Religious icons are, however, converted from neutral to threat. For the person troubled by aggressive thoughts towards children, churches and religious icons remain neutral (see also below in the discussion of obsessional content).

It is curious—but revealing—how frequently the potential 'victims' who feature in harm obsessions are helpless. Typically, the 'victims' are the elderly, the disabled, the very young. Probably this is so exactly because they are helpless; this makes the intrusive thought utterly immoral or repugnant, and hence, the affected person attaches even greater significance to these horrible obsessions. For example, 'If I have such repulsive, utterly unjustifiable horrible thoughts, then I must be totally immoral and dangerous'. There can be no more repugnant idea than injuring people who are helpless. This analysis is illustrated in a series of steps with accompanying examples (see Table 1.2). It is also worth noticing that people rarely (ever?) have harm obsessions about strong people who are well capable of defending themselves—there are no Arnold Schwartzenegger obsessions.

The relationship between catastrophic misinterpretations and the persistence of obsessions

The catastrophic misinterpretation placed on an unwanted intrusive thought increases the opportunities for the elicitation of obsession and hence the frequency of obsession increases. In a related manner, the catastrophic misinterpretation of the intrusive thought promotes persistence of the obsession. The particular obsession will persist for as long as the thoughts/images/impulses are interpreted as being of great personal significance. For example, if my obsessional images of violence are interpreted as meaning that I am a dangerously violent person, then this view of myself cannot be dismissed easily. The images are far too important and far too threatening to be ignored. One feels compelled to take action to reduce or to avoid the perceived danger, and these avoidance actions can be physical or mental. Actual avoidance or covert neutralization do provide temporary sanctuary or release. One moves to safer 'territory' or cancels the threat.

The significance of the obsession remains unaltered, however, and therefore the obsession will persist for as long as the person remains under threat (e.g. near children, in a kitchen containing sharp objects, etc.). Moving away from the threat, where and when this is possible, will temporarily interfere with the persistence of the obsession, only for it to return when the person is re-exposed to potentially threatening stimuli or internal sensations.

Again, by contrast, if the catastrophic misinterpretation is changed, reduced, or replaced, the internal and external cues are no longer interpreted as sources of threat. Now reduced to non-threatening cues, they can safely be dismissed or ignored. Unwanted intrusive thoughts that are regarded as insignificant will not persist.

Internal and external provocations of obsessions

Just as panic can be provoked when the person catastrophically misinterprets certain bodily sensations (Clark 1986), bodily sensations that occur in association with unwanted intrusive thoughts can also be catastrophically misinterpreted—say as confirmatory signs of an imminent loss of control, danger, and so forth. As mentioned earlier, if a person who suffers from unwanted intrusive thoughts of harming young children perceives himself to be trembling and sweating when in the presence of a child, he is likely to interpret the bodily signs as indicators of an impending loss of control and/or as signs of imminent aggression. With either interpretation, the occurrence of the bodily sensations in association with the obsession confirms the great importance of the unwanted intrusive thoughts: 'The fact that I am so upset here means that the thoughts must be important—why else would I tremble and sweat in the presence of unprotected children?'. The personal reactions appear to be inappropriate, perhaps dangerously inappropriate. The reactions are also out of context—perhaps what some patients mean when they reportedly complain that 'it doesn't feel right'. Another worry is that one's inability to control the unwanted thoughts can be taken as a sign that one cannot dependably control one's impulses to act, to harm others, say.

At this stage the person is faced with a choice. In trying to make sense of the fact that he repeatedly feels tense and trembling in the presence of young children, he can interpret this as meaningless nonsense or can interpret the feelings as signifying that he is a freak and unreliable in the presence of children.

More broadly, the very occurrence of the repugnant, unwanted, intrusive thoughts can be catastrophically misinterpreted as evidence of their significance (Salkovskis and Kirk 1997; Shafran 1997): 'The fact that I am repeatedly having these horrifying thoughts/images/impulses must mean that they are of special significance'. Very likely they are also interpreted to mean that the affected person is indeed different, perhaps a freak, evil, potentially dangerous, insane: 'Who else but a freak, psychopath, or insane person would keep having such unnatural and horrific impulses and thoughts?'. Incidentally, the significant misinterpretation of the very frequency of the intrusive unwanted thoughts (i.e. they must be important because I am having them so often), may help to explain the puzzle of those rare but baffling nonsensical obsessions that persist over long periods of time. It is possible, indeed, that they persist because the person interprets the intrusiveness of the nonsensical ideas, musical phrases, etc., as evidence of a hopeless irrationality that is of considerable significance, perhaps as the sign of impending mental illness, for example.

Of course it is essential for the affected person to conceal the fact of violent, obscene, unwanted intrusive thoughts from other people because 'they would draw the same conclusions about me as I have already done for myself' (e.g. 'If people discover that I am repeatedly having unnatural, dangerous and obscene impulses, they too will conclude that I am a freak or mentally ill or a psychopath').

For these reasons, the early and educational component of CBT (see below) can provide considerable relief for sufferers and prepare the ground for less catastrophic interpretations of their intrusive thoughts. Many patients obtain some useful and rapid relief on being informed (correctly) that virtually all people experience unwanted intrusive thoughts, and that the content of these nigh-universal unwanted intrusive thoughts is not too different from the content of clinical obsessions. Reading printed lists of the 'normal' obsessions can be a first step towards deflating the erroneously unique significance that the person attaches to his own intrusive thoughts—the experience of obsessions is not rare, nor is it a sign of freakishness or mental illness (see Toolkit). The difference between abnormal obsession and normal obsession lies not in the content as such (de Silva and Rachman 1997; Rachman and de Silva 1978) but in the significance that is attached to the experience, and in the distress and disablement that is consequent on this interpretation.

The content of obsessions

The particular content of obsessions can be deduced from the core of the present theory: that obsessions arise from the catastrophic misinterpretation of unwanted intrusive thoughts. We all experience unwanted intrusive thoughts but it is only a small minority of people who develop clinically significant obsessions. It is argued that this small group is vulnerable because of their pre-existing beliefs and cognitive biases. Moreover, the particular content of their obsessions will be determined by these very beliefs and biases. The unwanted intrusive thoughts that are subject to conversion into obsessions are those that have a particular significance for the affected person. The content of a person's obsessions, whether aggressive or sexual or blasphemous or a combination of these, will be determined not only by the general significance that they attach to intrusive thoughts, but also by the themes that are most important in the patient's system of values. If the person has very strong views about the need to behave compassionately, courteously, and gently, and rejects all violence ('I haven't an aggressive bone in my body'), the unwanted emergence of intrusive aggressive impulses is acutely unwelcome and distressing.

If one believes that it is essential to be consistently kind and helpful, the arrival of aggressive or violent impulses towards other people (especially if they are helpless) is particularly repugnant. This is a first step on the way to the emergence of an obsession, but it is not likely to proceed to the second and final stage unless the person makes a catastrophic misinterpretation of the meaning of the intrusive thought. It is perfectly possible for someone to be upset by an unwanted violent thought but to regard it as carrying little significance. In these instances, no obsession will be generated. In contrast, if the unwanted violent thoughts are interpreted as signifying that the person is potentially dangerous or evil, then the stage is set for the emergence of persisting obsessions.

A person of very high religious standards, particularly one who believes strongly that one should be as pure in thought as in deed, will be particularly upset by the unwanted intrusion of irreligious or sinful thoughts. A person who attaches especially strong value to conventionally acceptable sexual ideas and behaviour will be particularly upset by the unwanted appearance of obscene impulses, images, or thoughts. In general, it has been observed that the people who are prone to obsessional experiences are those who are of 'tender conscience' and those who are 'religiously quickened' (Rachman and

Table 1.3 The relationships between content, feelings, and behaviour

	Thought content	Interpretation	Typical feelings	Typical behaviour
1	Unacceptable, sexual, mean, blasphemy	Immoral	Guilt, rejection, fear of discovery	Conceal, put right, compensate, neutralize
2	Harmful, aggressive impulses/images re: elderly, disabled, young, injure, attack, cause accident.	Dangerous	Guilt, fear, inflated responsibility	Avoid, isolate, restrain, neutralize, check
3	Bizarre, out of context, puzzling	Going insane	Fear	Resist, conceal, seek help, medicate
4	Unacceptable, angry, extremist, shocking	Anti-social	Anxiety, anger	Conceal, resist, avoid

Hodgson 1980); and there are some notable historical examples of religious leaders who were tormented by blasphemous/obscene thoughts (e.g. John Bunyan, Martin Luther).

It is an unexplained oddity that there are three main themes of obsessions (harm, unacceptable sexual ideas, blasphemy), but some other unacceptable/immoral themes, such as avarice, rarely feature in obsessions.

The well-recognized connection between depression and obsessions (see Rachman 1997c) can be newly interpreted within the cognitive theory. Given the self-deprecatory ideas that form part of depression, people are especially vulnerable to attaching catastrophic personal significance to their intrusive thoughts when depressed. They already believe that they are immoral, useless, disturbed, guilty, and are therefore easy prey. It is a short and easy step to incorporate one's unwanted intrusive thoughts into this pre-existing negative self-view. The nasty thoughts do not intrude into neutral territory but, rather, are incorporated into a well-prepared personal vulnerability.

Given the person's vulnerability to attaching excessive importance to intrusions of particular content, it is possible to set up a rudimentary classification of the main types of thoughts involved: immoral, dangerous, anti-social, insane. It is postulated that the most common personal interpretations of such thoughts are: I am bad/dangerous; I will lose control and carry out the act; these irrational thoughts mean that I'm going crazy. A conceptual classification of these four main types with their associated behaviour, feelings and content, is set out in Table 1.3. Ultimately of course, this and similar classifications will need to be subjected to formal psychometric investigation and analysis.

Neutralization

People who experience obsessions frequently are inclined to take steps to 'put matters right', that is to neutralize the anticipated negative effects of the obsession or to neutralize the uncomfortable/guilty feelings engendered by the obsession (Salkovskis 1985). These attempts to undo or put right the obsession and its potential effects can be successful in the short run. There is clinical and experimental evidence showing that acts of neutralization are followed by significant reductions in anxiety/discomfort (Rachman *et al.* 1996). Most attempts at neutralization are not directly observable, and it is this very inaccessibility that has made them a difficult target in therapy. The overt forms of neutralization are more accessible and hence more tractable. However, we now have methods for converting the covert neutralizing activities into overt ones (Rachman *et al.* 1996).

Neutralization resembles compulsive behaviour but is not identical with it. Both neutralization and compulsion are commonly anxiety-reducing and it is believed that both of these activities are re-inforced and strengthened because they are successful in the short run (see Mowrer's two-factor theory: Mowrer 1939, 1960; Rachman and Hodgson 1980). However, not all acts of neutralization have compulsive qualities. Many acts of neutralization have the stereotypic and driven properties of the more common forms of compulsion, but other instances of neutralization are neither stereotypic nor driven by a compulsive urge to execute the neutralizing action, or even to do it repeatedly. Rather, many acts of neutralization are deliberately chosen tactics that are used selectively to deal with particular obsessions in certain circumstances (Rachman and de Silva 1978; Freeston and Ladouceur 1997). Unlike compulsions, these types of neutralizing act seldom give rise to resistance. On the contrary, the person intentionally adopts and uses them. They are tactics rather than compulsions.

In the long run, the use of neutralization is maladaptive because it helps to maintain the patient's belief that the act of neutralization was responsible for preventing the feared event from occurring and/or that without the neutralization the discomfort caused by the obsessions would have persisted. In these ways, neutralization shields the beliefs from disconfirmatory evidence.

If the feared event, say an obsessional impulse to harm an infant, is repeatedly anticipated but fails to occur, then the belief that one might carry out this type of aggressive act would, with frequent repetition, be weakened and finally disconfirmed. The sequence can be illustrated in these steps:

1 I have an intrusive unwanted impulse to harm an infant;

2 I believe that I may lose control and cause harm to infants;

3 but for therapeutic or spontaneous reasons I place myself in contact with infants;

4 however, I do not act on the impulse, I do not harm the infant;

5 after many repetitions of such exposures, my belief that I may act harmfully is disconfirmed;

6 the steady accumulation of this disconfirmatory evidence gradually weakens my belief that I may lose control and harm infants.

However, if instead of these planned exposures, I neutralize the unwanted impulse (and recall that neutralization is temporarily effective), then I am likely to believe that the act of neutralization helped to prevent the feared event: 'If I had not taken the precaution of neutralizing, then the feared event might have occurred'; 'If I hadn't left in time I might have molested that child'. The belief that I might carry out the obsessional impulse is shielded from disconfirmation. If anything, the repeated and temporarily effective use of neutralization will help to confirm the (competing) beliefs: 'I am so uncontrolled/dangerous that I must take steps to prevent myself from acting in a harmful manner', and/or also, 'If I had not neutralized the obsessional impulse, the feared event may well have occurred'.

It is assumed here that this cycle of:

obsession → neutralization → relief → confirmation of belief

is strengthened by repetition. It is further assumed that the cycle can be broken by repeatedly blocking the urge to neutralize.

If blocking is instituted, the affected person acquires two important pieces of information. First, he/she learns that the feared event does not occur, even if no neutralization precautions are taken. Secondly, he/she learns that the anxiety aroused by the obsession diminishes spontaneously—it declines, even in the absence of attempts at neutralization.

This new information can help to modify the inflated significance attached to the obsession. The obsession need no longer be interpreted as a premonitory sign of loss of control, or of danger. New information can also undermine the idea that the obsessions are of significance in revealing that the affected person is dangerous, insane, on the verge of losing control. Furthermore, learning that the anxiety dissipates spontaneously can help to weaken the inflated significance that is given to the obsession. The thoughts, impulses, or images are not so important that they must be corrected, put right, or neutralized; obsessions and their associated anxiety/discomfort fade away naturally, spontaneously. They are not so important that they must be dealt with, immediately and fully. They can safely be ignored or dismissed. They are 'noise' rather than meaningful signals.

Of course, neutralization is only one of several possible reactions to the experience of an obsession. The same reasoning, including the hypotheses and predictions, can be applied with minor modifications to other reactions, such as repeated avoidance behaviour. For example, 'I have harmful obsessions regarding children, and must therefore take care to avoid being alone with them'. The fact that no harmful acts actually occur is then ascribed to the precautionary avoidance behaviour, and the catastrophic misinterpretation of the obsession is left unchallenged and unchanged.

Catastrophic misinterpretations of obsessions can also trigger a sequence of self-sustaining stress in which a particular reaction to the obsession causes a paradoxical increase in the very obsession itself. Although the parameters of the phenomenon are still unclear, there is evidence that deliberate attempts to suppress particular unwanted thoughts can lead to a paradoxical increase in their frequency—the so-called 'white bear' effect (Wegner and Pennebaker 1993). For example, if people are instructed not to think about white bears, in many circumstances they will then experience a paradoxical increase in the number of such thoughts (e.g. Clark and Ball 1991; Salkovskis and Campbell 1994; Gold and Wegner 1995). From the present point of view, an inflated increase in the significance attached to an unwanted intrusive thought, such as an obsession, will lead to more vigorous and intense attempts to suppress such thoughts: 'They are so horrible and repugnant and dangerous that I must fight them off'. These attempts can produce an increase in the frequency of the obsession.

In contrast, it is predicted that a reduction in the catastrophic interpretation placed on the obsession will lead to fewer and less intense attempts to fight against the obsession. This in turn will be followed by a reduction in the frequency of the obsession. This specific prediction consists of three stages:

1 the catastrophic interpretation of the obsession is reduced;

2 there is an ensuing reduction in attempts to suppress the obsession;

3 there is a reduction in the frequency of the obsession.

Given that patients can misinterpret the frequency with which they experience the obsession as evidence of the importance of the obsession (Salkovskis 1985; Salkovskis and Kirk 1997; Shafran 1997, and see the case excerpt on p. 80), paradoxical increases in frequency that arise from attempts at suppression may actually strengthen the catastrophic misinterpretation themselves. A vicious circle is established:

1 These repugnant thoughts are highly significant for me.

2 I must suppress them.

3 They paradoxically increase in frequency.

4 The fact that I keep getting these repugnant thoughts means that they are indeed highly significant for me.

5 I must suppress them.

Responsibility

The concept of inflated responsibility introduced by Salkovskis (1985) refers to a tendency for people with OCD to feel an exaggerated sense of responsibility for actual, imagined, or anticipated misfortunes, to feel pivotally responsible for such misfortunes.

As described earlier, inflated responsibility can be a vulnerability factor and/or an interpretation placed on an event or thought (Salkovskis 1985; Obsessive Compulsive Cognitions Working Group 1997, 2001). In the present discussion, the same two properties of inflated responsibility can be discerned. People who are prone to feel exaggerated responsibility, especially for preventing misfortunes, are bound to be easily inclined to make catastrophic misinterpretations of their unwanted intrusive thoughts, particularly when the thoughts/impulses involve potential harm to others. They will also experience intense responsibility for the effects and/or immorality of their bad thoughts, as exemplified best in the cognitive bias of TAF: 'My harmful thought increases the probability that my friends/relatives will come to harm, perhaps be injured or even die'; 'I am responsible, I am to blame' (see Rachman 1993). The precise connections between inflated responsibility (both as a factor contributing to one's vulnerability to obsession and as a biased style of interpreting one's cognitions) and the mechanisms of obsessions remain to be established.

Who is vulnerable?

As with Clark's (1986) theory of panic, the people who are vulnerable (to obsessions) are those who are prone to make catastrophic misinterpretations (of the significance of their intrusive thoughts).

As a general background, people who are taught, or learn, that all of their value-laden thoughts are of significance, will be more prone to obsessions—as in particular types of religious beliefs and instruction. Striving to be moral, all of one's actions and thoughts must strive for virtue—moral perfectionism. Immoral thoughts are interpreted as comparable to, or even equivalent to, immoral actions. Some of the great religious leaders were subject to intrusive obsessions (see Rachman and Hodgson 1980). Plainly, not all people with highly elevated religious or moral standards suffer from abnormal obsessions. There must be additional contributory factors.

The proneness to use, or be led by, particular cognitive biases, is another vulnerability factor. TAF is a prime candidate here because of the assumed connection between the thought and the feared action/event. This bias also inflates one's sense of responsibility, and elevated responsibility is itself a vulnerability factor (Salkovskis 1985; Salkovskis and Kirk 1997).

Undoubtedly, depression increases one's vulnerability to obsessions (e.g. Ricciardi and McNally 1995), so this must be included as a risk factor for obsessions. It remains to be seen what the mechanism is—does depression promote obsessions by altering the way in which one interprets the intrusive thoughts, perhaps by giving the most pessimistic explanation? Here, Beck's (1976) theory of depression is relevant but the details will need to be worked out. Another factor is that in a state of depression, the person's self-evaluation is already negative (e.g. I am worthless, immoral) and, therefore, serious misinterpretations of the meaning of one's intrusive thoughts fall into well-prepared ground.

A fourth contributor is anxiety proneness itself, because it is known that anxiety-provoking materials, such as films, specific stressors, etc., increase the frequency of intrusive thoughts, the raw material out of which obsessions emerge. So people who react with anxiety to a wide range of stimuli/situations will experience many more intrusive thoughts, and if the significance of one or many of these thoughts is catastrophically misinterpreted, then obsessions take occupation.

At this stage then, at least four vulnerability factors can be postulated:

1 elevated moral standards;
2 particular cognitive biases;
3 depression;
4 anxiety.

None of these is novel, but in the present theory they are integrated and set out in a manner that invites direct testing. Research testing of the theory is in its early stages but the results are promising. For example, Purdon (2001) showed that when participants interpreted their thought recurrences as signifying unpleasant personal characteristics, or of foretelling misfortune, they reported increases in anxiety and a negative mood state.

Treatment implications

It follows from the theory that the most direct and satisfactory treatment of obsessions is to assist patients in the modification of the putatively causal catastrophic misinterpretations of the significance of their intrusive thoughts. Bluntly, if these misinterpretations are 'corrected', the obsessions should cease (see Rachman 1998).

As the treatment is focused on changing the misinterpretations of the significance of the intrusive thoughts, the first step is educational. Patients are informed that unwanted intrusive thoughts/images/impulses are commonplace, indeed nearly universal—a printed list of common examples is helpful here. Learning that obsession is a well-recognized problem helps to dissolve some guilt and anxiety, especially if the obsession has been concealed as a private secret fear and a cause for shame.

The second step is to inform them that intrusive thoughts, including their own obsessions, are not signs of some deep, concealed part of their character—they are not revealing of character. Moreover, some greatly admired public figures, such as Bunyan, have suffered from obsessions. Far more important than these uninvited, unwanted, fragmentary thoughts are the patient's personal history, achievements, values, standards, and conduct. These are what matter—these are the 'revealing' qualities of one's character.

The next stage is to collect a full account of the content of the obsessions and to discuss the content in a calm, dispassionate manner—as a clinical problem rather than as previously, a cause of shame, distress, and threat. Encouraging the patient to describe and then record the occurrence of the obsession, in a preferably boring and mechanical form, helps to detoxify the obsession, to change its significance.

The collection of this information is then used, in the usual way of cognitive therapy (e.g. Steketee 1994; Salkovskis 1999), as a basis for assessing the patient's interpretation of the obsession. As ever, the patient is encouraged to construct alternative interpretations of the intrusive thoughts and to match the available evidence for and against the original catastrophic significance and the alternatives (for excellent advice on changing the appraisals see Freeston *et al.* 1996). This may include behavioural experiments designed to collect new evidence that permits tests of the different interpretations.

The patient is encouraged at this stage to interpret the unwanted intrusive thoughts as 'noise' rather than as the true signal. The analogy of a radio can be helpful here—when a radio is off-station, we try to scan out the noise, the better to receive the true signal.

The avoidance behaviour that results from the obsessions is tackled in the usual way: encouraging the patients gradually and steadily to expose themselves to the anxiety-evoking situations (e.g. spending increasing amounts of time with children).

Cognitive therapists have yet to establish powerful methods for reducing cognitive biases, and, indeed, until recently there was pessimism about whether any such biases could be removed (e.g. Dawes *et al.* 1989). In the context of medical clinical reasoning, Arkes (1981) suggest the following tactics to minimize biases:

- avoid dichotomous judgments;
- take into account non-occurrences of events;
- consider the alternatives;
- collect disconfirmatory evidence;
- think Bayesian.

Some of these tactics can be adapted for the treatment of obsessions. Given the important role of inflated responsibility in OCD (Salkovskis 1985), and in obsessions in particular, the therapist should assist the affected patients to deflate this problem (see Salkovskis and Kirk 1997).

This combination of tactics should prove useful, but the focus on modifying the putative misinterpretations of the significance of the intrusive thoughts is maintained throughout.

The nature and measurement of 'significance'

The defining quality of the significance attached to intrusive thoughts is the person's belief that the thought (image, impulse) is meaningful and it is important; it is not trivial, it is not meaningless but is revealing about me. A second feature of this significance is that it is personalized, the thought is my own and it is especially important to me in particular: 'My recurrent images of committing incestuous acts with my young sister reveal that I, in particular, am deeply flawed and immoral'; 'My recurrent violent impulses to assault children reveal that I, in particular, am a potentially dangerous and evil person'. Third, the thought is alien to me, ego-alien. Fourth, the thought is believed to have potential consequences; it is not a mere passing thought bereft of any future. Fifth, the potential consequences are serious. There are unusual exceptions in which the obsession appears to be meaningless or the consequences are not unusually serious. Examples of nonsensical obsessions, such as recurrent and distressingly persistent advertisement jingles, can give rise to interpretations of serious mental illness (my mind is out of control, this is a sign of impending mental illness).

All of these interpretations of unwanted intrusive thoughts, and more to come, can and should be assessed. The thought/image/impulse can be rated on several dimensions:

- it is meaningful
- it is revealing about me
- it is important
- it is my thought

- it has special meaning for me
- the thought is alien to my values and beliefs
- it is personalized
- it has potential consequences
- these potential consequences are serious
- I have to do whatever I can to stop the thought (or its consequences)
- I have to take special care to avoid acting on the thought.

These are set out as for an assessment of a particular thought/image/impulse and, wherever possible, particularity should be pursued. Of course there will be instances in which a theme or cluster of several thoughts may need to be assessed.

Useful progress has been made by the international working group that was established to develop methods for assessing obsessive beliefs and obsessive interpetations of intrusive thoughts (Obsessive Compulsive Cognitions Working Group 1997, 2001; Frost and Steketee 2002).

Summary

Starting from the premise that unwanted intrusive thoughts are the basis of obsession, and encouraged by the finding that these thoughts are almost universally experienced, the behavioural theory of obsession was developed into a cognitive theory, based on the work of Clark and Salkovskis. It is postulated that obsessions are caused by catastrophic misinterpretations of the significance of one's unwanted intrusive thoughts. By deduction, any increase in such interpretations will produce or increase the obsessions. Similarly, any reduction in such misinterpretations will be followed by a reduction in obsessions.

CHAPTER 2

Background and rationale

Initial attempts to explain obsessions within the framework of behaviour therapy made little progress (Eysenck and Rachman 1965). At that time, the construal of obsessions was grounded in classical psychiatry and was strong on phenomenology but weak on aetiology (Lewis 1936, 1966; Jaspers 1963). Obsessions were regarded as qualitatively distinct, a form of pathological thinking, a 'pathology spot'. Obsessions were well described, as repugnant, intrusive thoughts that the person resisted, and they were separated from phenomena such as thought insertion, ideas of reference, feelings that one's thoughts were being manipulated by an outside force, and so forth. The pathological construal of obsessions (based on the two Rs—repugnance and resistance) assumed that we were dealing with a qualitatively different form of thinking, and this approach was not open to a psychological explanation, let alone a behavioural one. There was nothing in the academic approach to the psychology of thinking to cast light on this pathological form of thinking, and the behavioural clinicians had no tools to study thinking, pathological or normal. Explanations were attempted, but floundered so quickly that it was conceded that little progress could be expected unless obsessions were re-construed as extensions of the normal; in keeping with the general drift of behavioural psychology, the construal of unusual/disturbed behaviour as being pathological was challenged and replaced with the idea that abnormal behaviour lies at the far end of a normal continuum of behaviour. It is at the extreme end of normal. So obsessions were then re-construed as extreme manifestations of normal thinking—leading to the initially surprising recognition that everyone experiences unwanted, intrusive thoughts and that these closely resemble clinical obsessions in both form and content (Rachman 1971, 1976a).

Pursuing this re-construal, Rachman and de Silva (1978) attempted to find out whether obsessions do indeed resemble normal thinking. They tried to determine whether or not obsessions could be 'normalized' in this manner by studying eight obsessional patients and 124 non-clinical comparison subjects. It turned out that 'normal obsessions' are a common experience, described by the vast majority of the non-clinical subjects, as well as by the patients. Moreover, the form of the normal obsessions was indistinguishable from that of the clinical obsessions. The content of the unwanted, nasty, intrusive thoughts was remarkably similar in the clinical and non-clinical groups; so much so that when a large number of examples, drawn from the clinical and non-clinical respondents, were given to psychiatrists, psychologists, and psychiatric nurses to classify blindly, the results were conclusive—these experienced clinicians were unable to distinguish between the content of the clinical and non-clinical obsessions. However, the normal and abnormal obsessions did differ in important ways, including frequency, duration, intensity, and consequences. In a close replication carried out by Salkovskis and Harrison (1984), the results were confirmed (see also Niler and Beck 1989). In an extensive psychometric investigation, Thordarson (2001) also replicated the main findings and went on to demonstrate that the interrelationships between the thoughts and the interpretations placed on them were comparable in clinical and non-clinical groups. For example, even in non-obsessive compulsive disorder (OCD) comparison groups, the frequency and distress associated with negative intrusive thoughts is correlated with the way in which these thoughts are interpreted by the respondents. This correlation was unchanged, even when she partialled out the potential effects of depression. In general, her findings 'supported the idea of continuity between the experience of normal intrusive thoughts and clinical obsessions; that is, that clinical obsessions are an extreme form of normal intrusive thoughts' (p. 117).

The conclusion that obsessions are an extreme form of a universal phenomenon, namely that we all experience unwanted intrusive thoughts, runs contrary to the unexamined notion that we have full control over our daily thoughts. A belief in such control is difficult to reconcile with the considerable efforts that are required to control, direct, exclude, and edit our daily thoughts. One has only to consider the great difficulty that students encounter in trying to think about and concentrate on their studies. Only a small proportion of one's daily thoughts are the result of deliberate selection. Even that small proportion of our thoughts that is deliberately chosen does not necessarily move in the direction, or reach the conclusions, that we seek. Many of our thoughts, indeed the majority of them, appear to flow in and out and about without deliberate selection or direction, the so-called stream of consciousness. In this flow of intrusive thinking, a proportion is bound to be unwanted or even objectionable, and if the person interprets the objectionable thoughts as increasing the probability of a misfortune, or interprets the thoughts as having great personal and negative significance, then psychological problems can arise.

The major question to arise from the demonstration that unwanted intrusive thinking, including so-called normal obsessions, are commonplace, is the nature and cause of the shift from a normal intrusive thought to one of the extreme forms that are characteristic of clinical obsession. Why do the unwanted intrusive thoughts of everyday life sometimes develop into distressing and persistent obsessions? The germ of an idea was introduced 25 years ago, but not developed until many years later: 'So far from accepting the validity of the obsession, our . . . patients are told that most people experience unwanted, unacceptable intrusive thoughts, but that they rarely attach significance to these useless ideas and, therefore, dismiss them easily. The patients are encouraged to regard their obsessions as alien and useless and then taught how to detoxify them' (Rachman 1976a, p. 438). The enabling event that opened the door to a fresh attempt at explaining obsessions was the publication of Salkovskis's theoretical paper on a cognitive approach to obsession. He reasoned that 'the crucial cognitive element was not the intrusions (which were in any case, a universal phenomenon) but rather the meaning that the person attached to such intrusions. This way of conceptualizing obsessions has similar features to cognitive approaches to other anxiety problems, with the key differences arising from the consequences from the specific beliefs of the person concerned' (Salkovskis 1998, p. 37). He developed this original idea with great success, and also identified a sense of inflated responsibility as a key element in OCD.

Shortly after the publication of Salkovskis's original approach, Clark (1986) published his landmark cognitive theory of panic, in which he argued that panic is caused by a catastrophic misinterpretation of certain bodily sensations. This theory too was successfully developed and covered a wide range of panic phenomena, including the triggers of an episode, the factors that maintain a proneness to panic, a rational derivation of therapy, and so forth. By combining the panic theory and Salkovskis's unfolding explanation of the role of appraisals in OCD, the specific theory of obsession was developed. As with the panic theory, elaborations of the theory of obsession have lead to hypotheses regarding the proneness to obsession, the triggers that set them off, and the factors that maintain them. In each instance, the ensuing therapy is derived directly from the theory. Following the model of Clark's theory of cognitive theory of panic, it is argued that obsessions are caused by a catastrophic misinterpretation of the personal significance of specific unwanted intrusive thoughts.

The importance of thoughts

Support for the view that the patient's interpretation of their intrusive thoughts may play a role in the causes and/or maintenance of obsession comes from some of the interim findings of the international group that is engaged in the development of methods for assessing OCD cognitions (Obsessive

Compulsive Cognitions Working Group 1997, 2001; Frost and Steketee 2002). The Group constructed two scales: one to measure obsessional beliefs, and the other to measure the person's interpretation of their intrusive thoughts. The two scales have been tested on 17 samples, drawn from seven countries. The latest findings, drawn from 257 OCD respondents, 104 anxiety disorder controls, and 85 community controls, showed that the OCD group had significantly higher scores than the anxiety controls on beliefs about the importance of their thoughts, the need to control their thoughts, and on responsibility. The correlation between scores on the importance of thoughts subscale and the control of thoughts subscale is to be expected. Why would one strive to control an unimportant thought? It is the important thoughts that call for control.

Producing suitably reliable, discriminating, and precise scales has proved to be a difficult task, and statistical and other problems have emerged. For example, the high correlation between the two scales raises doubts about whether they have yet succeeded in separating out the beliefs and the interpretations, or even whether such a division is possible. The composition of the OCD group, based on the DSM psychiatric diagnostic system, makes no distinction between the broad definition of obsessions, which includes most types of preoccupying thoughts, even those that dwell on contamination fears, etc., and the repugnant and resisted classical obsessions. In order to sharpen the testability of the present approach to obsessions, which rests on the person's interpretation of repugnant intrusive thoughts, two additional steps are required. It follows from the cognitive theory that there should be specifiable differences between groups of patients with classical obsessions and patients with only the broad form of obsessions, and even greater differences between those with classical obsessions and patients with OCD that does not include obsessions. In addition, because of the critical importance attached to the patient's specific, idiosyncratic interpretations of their unwanted intrusive thoughts, reliable means for assessing these subtle individual differences need to be developed.

Thordarson (2001) carried out a thorough psychometric investigation on a group of 69 patients diagnosed with OCD, 39 community adult participants without any clinical disorder, and a second comparison group of 198 students. The respondents completed scales measuring obsessional compulsive problems, obsessional beliefs, and their interpretations of their intrusive thoughts (these last two scales were adapted from those constructed by the international working group referred to above). Most of the analyses of the relationship between importance of thoughts and obsessions were concentrated on the data collected on the importance of thoughts subscale of the interpretation inventory prepared by the working group. Typical items from this subscale include the following:

'Having this unwanted thought means I will act on it'; 'Thinking this thought could make it happen'; 'Having this thought means that I am weird or abnormal'; 'Having this intrusive thought means that I am a terrible person'.

Thordarson's non-clinical respondents reported that they did indeed experience unwanted intrusive thoughts, and the content of these thoughts was similar to that described by the patients with OCD. However, the patient group attached significantly greater importance to their intrusive thoughts, had more of them than did the comparison groups, and also found them to be more distressing—recalling the early findings on abnormal and normal obsessions described above. Among the patients, the correlation between importance of thoughts and obsessions was 0.50, which was significant at the 0.001 level. This correlation was unaffected when Thordarson partialled out responsibility for thoughts, control of thoughts, and scores on the Beck Depression Inventory. In a focused analysis conducted within the group of patients with OCD, she compared the scores given by those respondents who experienced repugnant obsessions with the scores returned by patients with OCD who did not experience repugnant obsessions. The patients for whom repugnant obsessions were a major problem, had a significantly higher score on the importance of their beliefs about their own thoughts than did the patients who were without repugnant obsessions, 'Suggesting that the beliefs in the importance of thoughts are particularly relevant for OCD sufferers with repugnant obsessions rather than other types of symptoms' (Thordarson 2001, p. 110). These findings are consistent with the cognitive theory of obsession. Further tests will require the development of more sharply focused scales to measure the repugnant unwanted, intrusive thoughts, to measure resistance, and, ultimately, the theory must be subjected to precise experimental analyses.

Inflated responsibility

Salkovskis (1985) attached particular importance to the role of inflated responsibility in the development and persistence of OCD: 'Normal intrusive thoughts and obsessions differ not in the occurrence or controllability of these thoughts, but in the way in which obsessional patients interpret intrusions as an indication that they may be responsible for harm or its prevention' (p. 39). He went on to argue that only those people who have an enduring tendency to misinterpret their own mental activity as indicating personal 'responsibility' will experience the pattern of discomfort and neutralizing activities of OCD. For example, when a particular thought is interpreted as indicating that the person 'has become responsible for harm to himself or herself or others, then the occurrence and the content of the thought becomes both a source of discomfort and an imperative signal for action that is intended to neutralize the thought and the potentially harmful consequence of its occurrence' (p. 41). The meaning of the thoughts, in terms of responsibility, is what distinguishes obsessional cognitions from depressed or anxious cognitions. The patients' attempts to control their thoughts or their consequences have the paradoxical effect of strengthening the obsessions, and Salkovskis (1998) draws particular attention to the adverse affects of thought monitoring, thought suppression, and neutralizing. Interestingly, it had been suggested that excessive responsibility plays a part in compulsive checking; for example, 'The most notable characteristics of obsessional checkers appear to include the following—an expressed fear of causing harm to themselves or others . . . checking mostly in the home . . . less intense when responsibility is diminished' (Rachman 1976b, p. 273). And again, 'Increases in responsibility will result in increased checking behaviour' (p. 275).

A range of psychometric and experimental evidence is consistent with Salkovskis's emphasis on the role of responsibility appraisals (see Rachman and Shafran 1998). In an experimental analysis, Lopatka and Rachman (1995) predicted that changes in perceived responsibility are followed by corresponding changes in the urge to check compulsively. The prediction was tested on 30 OCD patients whose major problem was compulsive checking. They agreed to participate in the experiment conducted in their own homes (in order to avoid the confounding caused by a loss of responsibility for actions carried out in the detached and remote environment of the laboratory). Each patient was asked to carry out a selected domestic task that provoked checking—under two counterbalanced conditions. In one condition they were asked to retain responsibility for the task and its consequences, but in the critical condition they were requested to transfer responsibility to the experimenter during and after carrying out the identical task. Even though the transfer of responsibility proved to be difficult in a number of cases because of the patient's resistance to divesting even a small part of their responsibility, albeit temporarily, the manipulation was successful in the main. As predicted, the deliberate reduction in responsibility was followed by a significant decline in discomfort and in the urge to carry out the compulsive checking (see Figs 2.1 and 2.2). A full account of the cognitive theory of compulsive checking is given in Rachman (2002a, 2002b).

Responsibility has also been manipulated by a number of related techniques. For example, Shafran (1997) did so indirectly by varying the presence or absence of the experimenter during a compulsive checking task. The manipulation was successful in that the perceived responsibility for threat was greater when the subject was alone than when the experimenter was present. In the high-responsibility condition, estimates of the urge to neutralize, discomfort, and probability of threat, were all significantly greater than in the

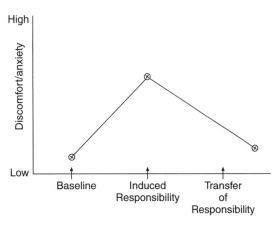

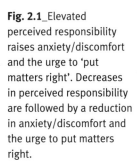

Fig. 2.1_Elevated perceived responsibility raises anxiety/discomfort and the urge to 'put matters right'. Decreases in perceived responsibility are followed by a reduction in anxiety/discomfort and the urge to put matters right.

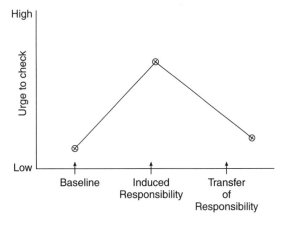

Fig. 2.2_The transfer of responsibility is followed by a reduction in discomfort and in the urge to check (adapted from Lopatka and Rachman 1995).

low-responsibility condition. The experimental findings on the effects of the deliberate reduction of responsibility provide a basis for therapeutic attempts to reduce inflated responsibility, especially by arranging for a transfer of responsibility (see Chapter 7).

Results from experiments and psychometric studies of this kind support the conclusion that OCD phenomena are much influenced by a person's perceived responsibility for threat. In the case of obsession, inflated responsibility is particularly noticeable when people are prone to the cognitive bias of thought–action fusion (TAF). As described below, when patients feel that their thoughts can have an adverse influence on other people, even cause them actual harm, their sense of responsibility is inevitably elevated.

In this context the recent uncovering of cognitive biases in the thinking of patients with OCD assumes considerable importance.

Cognitive biases in OCD

It has been observed that some patients with OCD tend to engage in magical thinking, defying or leaping over conventional rules of reasoning. The work of Tversky and Kahnemann (1974) on cognitive biases opened the door to an intensive investigation of these biases (see Nisbett and Ross 1980), and it later emerged that patients with OCD are prone to some distinctive cognitive biases.

As described earlier, the best established cognitive bias is TAF, in which thoughts and actions are entwined and people feel that their thoughts, especially the nasty ones, can affect external events (probability bias), and/or the morality bias in which an objectionable intrusive thought is regarded as being morally equivalent to the implied action.

One patient suffering from compulsive checking and obsessions went to extreme lengths to ensure that he never went to bed in a state of advanced tiredness. This tactic was intended to reduce the threat of dying in his sleep. He feared that if he allowed himself to fall into a very deep sleep, he might never wake up. The patient denied that the therapist was under similar threat because the therapist did not believe that he would be in danger from a deep sleep. The patient explained that he was in danger precisely because he held the belief that, for him, deep sleep could be fatal. He insisted that his thoughts increased the actual probability of dying. On further exploration, it emerged that he endorsed a number of beliefs in which thought and action were psychologically intertwined. Enquiries with other patients suffering from OCD revealed that this type of fusion was not uncommon and the phenomenon was labelled 'thought–action fusion' (Rachman 1993).

The majority of people reject or resist this form of psychological fusion and successfully distinguish between their uninvited, repugnant thoughts and their actions. They readily dismiss the thoughts and regard them as mental flotsam. This is not the case for people who have OCD. People who accept the view that immoral thoughts are equivalent to sinful acts (a view consistent with some religious thinking), nevertheless distinguish between these socially sanctioned fusions and their personal, idiosyncratic fusions. The TAF that is implicated in obsessional disorders is based on strongly held private beliefs, in contrast to fusions that are socially sanctioned and commonly shared.

A third cognitive bias is the belief that the probability of a misfortune occurring is greatly increased when one is in a responsible position (Lopatka and Rachman 1995): 'If I am left in charge, if I am responsible, then something is certain to go wrong'. This cognitive bias is disruptive but remains to be studied in fine detail.

A scale to measure both forms of TAF was constructed and given to two large groups of students (Shafran *et al.* 1996). It was found to be a coherent scale and the two forms of TAF were distinguishable, and significantly related to, obsessionality. Consistent results were reported by Amir *et al.* (2001), and by Emmelkamp and Aardema (1999) who concluded that TAF is 'related to most forms of obsessive compulsive behaviour' (p. 139). Rassin *et al.* (2001) found evidence of TAF in patients with OCD and in other forms of anxiety disorder, and also showed that TAF scores decreased after therapy. This is an encouraging finding and is in keeping with the demonstration by Zucker *et al.* (2002) that, among students with elevated TAF scores, a simple educational intervention was corrective. The cognitive bias of TAF certainly can contribute to the persistence and distress of the obsessions, and deserves therapeutic attention, but notwithstanding the encouraging results of Rassin and of Craske, TAF can be as resilient as other cognitive biases (Nisbett and Ross 1980) and defy easy reduction. Attempts to help the patient diminish his belief that he might die in his sleep exactly because he believed that he was vulnerable, were only of slight value. His degree of conviction declined from 99 to 80%. At this stage, the best way to tackle TAF is by a combination of education and behavioural experiments (see Chapter 5).

A tendency towards TAF can be a predisposing factor in OCD because personally significant intrusive thoughts, especially those pertaining to harming others, may be interpreted to mean that the danger to the person featured in the thought has been raised, and the patient is responsible for this increased threat. Other predisposing factors include perfectionism (Shafran and Mansell 2001; Frost and Steketee 2002), the cognitive bias regarding responsibility and probability of harm, anxiety and depression (Ricciardi and McNally 1995).

Thought suppression and neutralization

Resistance to objectionable intrusive thoughts can take a variety of forms but the most common appears to be thought suppression, in which the person makes strenuous efforts to refrain from having the unwanted thought (Freeston and Ladouceur 1997). This is variously described by patients as thought blocking or thought distraction or thought blanketing. There is, however, some evidence that these various attempts at suppressing unwanted thoughts can cause a paradoxical increase in their intrusiveness or frequency (see Salkovskis 1998; Purdon 1999). As the evidence is inconsistent, strong conclusions cannot be made at present. There have been some clear demonstrations of a paradoxical increase in the 'forbidden' thought when the person attempts to suppress it. A delayed rebound effect, in which the intrusive thought becomes more frequent and more prominent after a period of thought suppression, has also been observed. Purdon and Clark (2000) found that a person's mood can deteriorate after thought suppression. If such paradoxical consequences of thought suppression occur with regularity, it is easy to see how they might make an unfortunate contribution to an exacerbation of the problem. Freeston and Ladouceur (1997) collected examples of the tactics that patients use to deal with their obsessions, and most of them were, alas, useless. High on the list of the useless were thought stopping and internal debates. Relaxation was found to be helpful, as was a devaluation of the significance of the thought.

It has been argued that neutralization purchases a temporary relief at the price of conserving and even consolidating the misinterpretations that lie at the root of the obsessional problem. When attempts to block the unacceptable thought fail, it is common to resort to neutralizing the feared consequences of the nasty thought. Such neutralization can take a variety of forms, such as those described by Shafran and others (1996). These attempts at neutralization include forming a counter-thought, carrying out a neutralizing action, attempting to dampen the thought and its effects by engaging in distracting activities, by avoidance behaviour, and so forth. In an attempt to make the internal neutralizing activities manifest and, therefore, open to experimental analyses, Shafran et al. (1996) recruited a number of students who had returned high scores on a questionnaire designed to measure proneness to TAF. In an attempt to discover whether neutralization does indeed resemble overt compulsions, 63 subjects were asked to write a sentence that would evoke anxiety. The sentences involved possible harm coming to a friend or relative. After completing the sentence, subjects were asked to rate their anxiety, responsibility, guilt, and the likelihood of harm occurring. The subjects were then instructed to immediately neutralize or to delay for 20 min before doing so. The subjects who were asked to neutralize immediately, reported prompt reductions in their adverse feelings. Subjects who were asked to delay any attempts at neutralization, reported an equally substantial reduction in adverse feelings, such as anxiety, at the end of the 20-min delay period. This experiment showed that neutralizing produces a prompt decrease in discomfort, but also that the discomfort will decline naturally, without any attempt to dampen it. This spontaneous, but relatively slow decline in discomfort, resembles the natural decay curve that is observed in urges to carry out compulsive acts. If compulsive urges are inhibited they undergo a slow natural decline, and now it appears that a similar process operates for urges to neutralize unacceptable, unwanted thoughts (see Fig. 2.3).

Given the prompt relief achieved by immediate neutralization, these attempts to cancel out the effects of thoughts about harm probably persist because they are at least temporarily successful. In this respect as well, they resemble compulsions (Rachman et al. 1996).

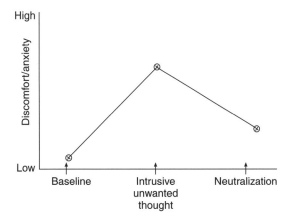

Fig. 2.3_Neutralization produces a prompt reduction in discomfort (adapted from Rachman *et al.* 1996).

Summary

To sum up, many unanswered questions remain but the trend of the evidence is encouraging. It has been established that having unwanted intrusive thoughts is indeed a common, normal experience. There is a remarkable continuity between unwanted intrusions and obsessions, including common content and form. However, the obsessions are more frequent, more persistent, and more distressing than other intrusions.

The hypothesis that patients with obsessions attach excessive importance to their intrusive thoughts is supported by psychometric and clinical evidence. The findings of the international working group also indicate that patients with OCD over-interpret the significance of their intrusive thoughts, and presumably those patients who are tormented by obsessions are especially prone to these over-interpretations.

There is growing evidence that patients with OCD are burdened with, and greatly influenced by, inflated responsibility. This influence extends to a responsibility for their unwanted intrusive thoughts, notably in the form of cognitive biases such as TAF. The hypothesis that the catastrophic misinterpretation of intrusive thoughts is the causal spark that transforms the unwanted thoughts into obsession, presents an experimental challenge, and has yet to be tested directly.

CHAPTER 3

Assessment procedures

Any person offered this course of cognitive treatment for obsessions should already have completed a general psychological assessment, and received a diagnosis of obsessive-compulsive disorder (OCD). It can be assumed further that the primary or sole problem of the OCD is obsession. In most cases of OCD, the initial assessment will have been carried out by a clinical psychologist, psychiatrist, or family doctor. This assessment generally consists of a clinical interview, supported by psychometric testing and/or referral on to a specialist in anxiety disorders. The two most commonly used structured interview methods for assessing OCD are the Yale Obsessive-Compulsive Scale (Y-BOCS) (Goodman *et al.* 1989), and the Anxiety Disorders Interview Schedule (ADIS-IV) (Brown *et al.* 1994). The two interviews are extremely useful but serve different purposes. The ADIS-IV screens for the presence of any anxiety disorder, including OCD. The Y-BOCS is a specialized instrument designed to determine the presence of OCD, its main features, severity, and consequences. For the treatment of obsessions, preliminary assessment by means of the Y-BOCS is preferred to the ADIS-IV. The ADIS-IV consists of several 'modules', each of which assesses a different anxiety disorder. Modules for assessing related disorders (e.g. depression, substance dependence), as well as screening questions for psychotic thoughts and behaviour, are included.

The Y-BOCS consists of an initial checklist of obsessional thoughts and compulsions, but the obsessions assessed by the Y-BOCS cover a broader range than the types of obsessions that are the focus of this manual. In keeping with the DSM, the Y-BOCS covers a wide range of persistent thoughts and includes as obsessions any recurrent thoughts that are preoccupying, such as those pertaining to compulsive cleaning, checking, etc., even if the thoughts lack the repugnant, immoral, objectionable qualities of classical obsessions and even in the absence of resistance. For example, recurrent and preoccupying thoughts about whether a situation is or is not contaminated are classed as obsessions, as are repeated thoughts about whether one has washed away all of the contaminants. Thoughts of this type are seldom resisted. Notwithstanding, the obsessions subscale of the Y-BOCS is a useful index of classical obsessions and should be included in pre- and post-treatment assessment.

Guided by the initial checklist, the patient and assessor agree on several target obsessions and compulsions, which are then rated on scales that assess frequency, distress, resistance, and so on. The Y-BOCS gives a total score, and separate scores for obsessions and compulsions.

Specialized assessments for the present treatment build on the initial assessment material but then take a more specific course. Given the emphasis on reducing/replacing the patient's catastrophic misinterpretations of their unwanted intrusive thoughts, the thrust of the specialized assessments is on the pre-, post-, and in-course assessments of the person's interpretations of their thoughts. Naturally, the therapist and patient also need to measure the broader effects of the treatment on anxiety, discomfort, avoidance, occupation, and so on. Here the therapist has a choice among the various instruments available; however, the indispensable, core assessments must address the nature and personal interpretations of the obsessions as such. For ordinary clinical use, an abbreviated assessment is sufficient. Given a prior diagnosis of OCD, the therapist can use the specialized scales, plus the Beck depression inventory (BDI), the obsessive-compulsive inventory (OCI), and the Y-BOCS self-report scales. In due course, the scales being developed by the Obsessive Compulsive Cognitions Working Group may be added.

For the specific assessment of obsessions, a specially constructed semi-structured interview is carried out (see Toolkit form 1). It is designed to collect information about the content and frequency of the obsessions, the triggers, safety behaviour, and maintaining conditions, as well as the personal significance that the patient attributes to the obsessions. Illustrative answers are shown in Toolkit form 1(a).

Toolkit form 1(a): Semi-structured interview on obsessions

1. Give me a full description of each of the troubling thoughts that keep coming into your mind against your wishes (quote patient's exact words whenever possible).

   (a) *e.g. I will lose control and stab my brother*

   (b)

   (c)

2. When, and how often, do you have each (a), (b), and (c)?

   e.g. several times per week

3. What sets them off? (a), (b), and (c)?

e.g. sight of sharp knives, being alone with my brother especially in the kitchen

Was there a particular moment/event when they began?

4. Do they affect:

(a) your concentration? *e.g. interfering*

(b) your mood? *e.g. make me feel miserable*

(c) your work? *e.g. minimally*

5. How do you attempt to deal with them?

e.g. try to argue against it

e.g. try to distract myself

e.g. avoid my brother

5a. Do you resist them? What will happen if you do not resist them?

e.g. yes, I might lose control, I might kill him

6. What helps you to deal with the thoughts?

e.g. distraction, company

7. What fails to help you deal with the thoughts?

e.g. arguing with myself, telling myself to stop the thoughts

8. Why do you think these thoughts began in the first place?

e.g. under stress at school

8a. Did you keep them secret—if so why?

e.g. yes, I am extremely ashamed of myself. people will think that I am a homicidal maniac

9. Have you told anyone else about these thoughts? (details please)

e.g. no one

10. How did they react?

e.g. N/A

11. Why do the thoughts keep coming back?

e.g. because I have a mental illness

12. Do these thoughts tell you anything about yourself—what kind of person you are?

e.g. I am an aggressive, dangerous person

13. Has it changed the way you behave towards other people?

e.g. keep away from others

14. Has it changed the way other people behave towards you?

e.g. can't say

15. What exactly will happen (apart from anxiety/discomfort) if you stop trying to cancel out the thoughts, block them, or fight against them?

e.g. I will lose control

16. Do you keep a close watch on these thoughts? Do you constantly monitor them?

e.g. no

> **16a.** What exactly will happen if you stopped monitoring the thoughts in this way?
>
> *e.g. N/A*

17. Have you ever acted out one of these thoughts? (details please)

e.g. never

18. Have these thoughts ever made you feel crazy, or about to go crazy? (details please)

e.g. yes, often, I may lose control

19. Have you ever felt that you might lose control and do something dangerous or weird? (details please)

e.g. yes, often

20. Do the thoughts make you feel that you cannot be trusted?

e.g. yes, definitely

21. If your thoughts are about harming other people, do they focus on particular people?

e.g. my brother mostly

22. Why do they focus on these particular people?

e.g. can't say why

23. Have you ever had similar harmful thoughts about any strong and confident person?

e.g. no

24. Most obsessions fall into one of three categories—aggressive thoughts, unacceptable sexual thoughts, and anti-religious thoughts—which group do your obsessions fall into?

e.g. aggressive

25. Why don't you have obsessions about the other categories?

e.g. can't say

26. Do your obsessions make you feel:
   (a) bad, wicked, or evil? *e.g. yes*
   (b) crazy or weird? *e.g. yes*
   (c) untrustworthy or dangerous? *e.g. yes*
   (d) other?

27. Are your thoughts related to your moods? Good moods or bad moods?

e.g. bad moods

28. After an upsetting event, do you spend a lot of time going over and over what happened and why?

e.g. yes, to sort it out in my mind

29. Have you ever received treatment for these distressing thoughts? If yes, when and where?

e.g. yes, medication, for two years

30. What were the effects? Why did it help, or fail to help you?

e.g. helped a little

Box 3.1 Assessments for treatment

Semi-structured interview: used at pre- and post-treatment, and at follow-up
Personal significance of thoughts: used at the start of each treatment session
Daily recording of unwanted, intrusive thoughts
Obsessional activity (patient): used at the start of each session
Obsessional activity (therapist-rated): used at the start of each session
Y-BOCS, especially the obsessions subscale: pre-, post-treatment, and follow-up
Obsessive-compulsive inventory (OCI)
Thought–action fusion (TAF) scale
Beck depression inventory (BDI)

Obsessive-compulsive inventory (OCI)

It is advisable to supplement the semi-structured interview with a self-report psychometric scale. One of the most widely used is the Maudsley obsessional compulsive inventory (MOCI) (Hodgson and Rachman 1977), which consists of 30 items and yields a total score plus two factor-scores (checking and cleaning). This scale was constructed when the main focus of treatment was on the observable OCD behaviour, namely checking and washing. For the measurement of obsessions, a modern scale such as the OCI (Foa *et al.* 1998b) is preferred. The OCI consists of 42 items (rated for both frequency and distress), which yield a total score and seven subscale scores. The reliability and validity are satisfactory. The inclusion of items assessing obsessions is an advance and makes it appropriate for the present therapy protocol.

Obsessional activity

When treatment begins, the patient is asked at the beginning of each session about the nature and amount of any obsessions experienced in the previous week—for this purpose, use Toolkit form 4: Measure of obsessional activity.

Personal significance scale

In order to assess and guide the course of therapy, it is essential to measure repeatedly: (i) the personal significance of the obsessions; and (ii) the amount of obsessional activity per week and the degree of distress it causes.

For this purpose the Personal significance scale is given at the beginning of each session (Toolkit form 2). Originally this scale was given at the beginning and end of each session, but so little immediate change occurred that we deleted the end of session administrations. It is best to use this scale at the start of each session, and in this way the therapist can track any changes in the patient's interpretation of their intrusive thoughts; it is an important index of change. The measurement of obsessional activity is completed by the patient at the start of each session and the therapist version is completed at the end of each session. The perspectives and appraisals of the patient and therapist tend to be similar but not identical, and hence both are needed.

The Personal significance scale consists of 26 questions, all of which are rated on a 10 cm visual analogue scale. The purpose of the questions is to gauge the personal significance that the person attaches to the unwanted intrusive thoughts. The expectation is that these interpretations will move in a more realistic direction during treatment, and, hopefully, key questions such as 'Do these thoughts reveal your true character?', 'Are these thoughts very significant?' will shift towards zero. The scale has four buffer questions: numbers 3 (original), 5 (imaginative), 13 (artistic), and 16 (sociable), and these can be ignored by the therapist. Illustrative answers are given in Toolkit form 2(a).

Toolkit form 2(a): Personal significance scale

Please read the following statements carefully and make a mark anywhere on the line to show the extent to which you agree with each statement.
Specific thoughts, images: *e.g. making an obscene gesture to a small child*

1. Are these thoughts all nonsense or are they significant for you?

not at all significant   somewhat significant   extremely significant

2. Do these thoughts reveal something important about you?

not at all important   somewhat important   extremely important

3. Are these thoughts a sign that you are original?

```
not at all            somewhat            very original
```

4. Do these thoughts mean that you might lose control and do something awful?

```
not at all            possibly            definitely
```

5. Do these thoughts mean that you are an imaginative person?

```
not at all imaginative    somewhat imaginative    extremely imaginative
```

6. Do these thoughts mean that you might go crazy one day?

```
not at all likely        somewhat likely        very likely
```

7. Is it important for you to keep these thoughts secret from most or all of the people you know?

```
not at all important    somewhat important    extremely important
```

8. Do these thoughts mean that you are a sensitive person?

```
not at all sensitive    somewhat sensitive    extremely sensitive
```

9. Do these thoughts mean that you are a dangerous person?

```
not at all dangerous    somewhat dangerous    definitely dangerous
```

10. Do these thoughts mean that you cannot be trusted?

```
completely trustworthy    somewhat trustworthy    not at all trustworthy
```

11. Would other people condemn or criticize you if they knew about your thoughts?

not at all	somewhat	definitely

12. Do these thoughts mean that you are really a hypocrite?

not at all	somewhat	definitely

13. Do these thoughts mean that you have an artistic talent?

not at all	somewhat	definitely

14. Would other people think that you are crazy or mentally unstable if they knew about your thoughts?

not at all	somewhat	definitely

15. Do these thoughts mean that one day you may actually carry out some actions related to the thoughts?

not at all likely	somewhat likely	very likely

16. Do these thoughts mean that you enjoy company?

not at all	somewhat	definitely

17. Do these thoughts mean that you are a bad, wicked person?

not at all	somewhat	definitely

18. Do you feel responsible for these thoughts?

not at all	somewhat	definitely

19. Do you feel that it is important for you to cancel out or block the thoughts?

not at all important	somewhat important	extremely important

20. Would other people think that you are a bad, wicked person if they knew about your thoughts?

not at all	somewhat	definitely

21. Do you think that you should avoid certain people or places because of these thoughts?

not at all	somewhat	definitely

22. Do these thoughts mean that you are weird?

not at all	somewhat	definitely

23. Do these thoughts mean something else? Please give details:

not at all	somewhat	definitely

24. Should you fight against and resist these thoughts?

not at all	somewhat	definitely

25. What caused your thoughts to occur when they started?

e.g. can't say for sure

26. Why do these thoughts keep coming back?

e.g. I'm weird

Patients can also keep a simple daily record of their unwanted intrusive thoughts. The Daily record (Toolkit form 5), covers the frequency, duration, intrusiveness, and distress caused by the thoughts.

Thought–action fusion (TAF) scale

As a guide to treatment, and also for research purposes, the 19-item self-report TAF scale (Shafran *et al.* 1996) is used. It provides a total score indicating the proneness to this cognitive bias, plus two subscores pertaining to probability TAF ('My thoughts increase the probability of a misfortune occurring') and to moral equivalence ('My thoughts are as morally objectionable as the relevant act'). (See Toolkit form 7.)

Beck depression inventory (BDI)

Given the common association between OCD and depression, and specifically between obsession and depression, a measure of depression is necessary. There are many scales to choose from and the widely used BDI serves well. The revised version, consisting of 21 items, is of satisfactory reliability and validity. Users can obtain the necessary information from the Center for Cognitive Therapy (telephone (1)-215-898-4100 or (1)-215-898-4102), 1 Belmont Ave., Bala Cynwyd, Pennsylvania, U.S.A. 19004).

Behavioural tests

In those cases where avoidance behaviour is prominent and contributing importantly to the problem, the use of a set of behavioural-avoidance tests is advisable. A list of avoidances is compiled and the most manipulable and relevant are selected for the tests (e.g. knives, sharp objects, supermarkets). The tests are carried out in the conventional way by observing the degree and extent of the patient's avoidance of specific objects or situations. In each case, the patient is asked to approach as close as possible to the object/situation and to rate their anxiety at the closest approximation. At the completion of treatment, little or no avoidance/anxiety should remain. The behavioural tests are an important assessment measure.

At various points in assessment, such as the behavioural tests, and in therapy, it is useful to have a simple measure of anxiety, and for this purpose, the commonly used fear thermometer is employed. The patient is asked to rate their anxiety on a 0–100 scale, where 0 = calm/no anxiety and 100 = terrified/extreme anxiety.

Thoughts about thoughts

Purdon and Clark (1999), among others, have correctly drawn attention to the importance of the patient's thoughts about their thoughts, the so-called meta-cognitions involved in obsession. It is argued here that the person's beliefs about, and especially their interpretations of, their unwanted intrusive thoughts are critical. As mentioned, an international working group has constructed a meta-cognitive scale for OCD, the obsessive beliefs questionnaire, and an accompanying scale for assessing the patient's interpretations of intrusions inventory (Obsessive Compulsive Cognitions Working Group 1997, 2001). The final versions of these two scales will be a valuable addition to the assessment of patients with OCD, and of particular relevance to the present theory and treatment procedures.

CHAPTER 4

Treatment—stage 1

The treatment takes place in two stages. The first stage is informative and educational. The second stage is the modification of the patients' maladaptive interpretations. Depending on the complexity, severity, and duration of the disorder, approximately 8–12 weekly sessions are required.

It is important to bear in mind that cognitive sessions often instigate a process of change that evolves slowly. Therapists who are accustomed to seeing fears reduce during exposure sessions, in front of them, are inclined to expect a similar immediacy during sessions that dwell on cognitive processes. More often than not, in cognitive behaviour therapy for obsessions, the changes evolve over a period of weeks, and are profoundly influenced by external events that occur between sessions. The emerging cognitive changes are shaped and consolidated by these events, and hence the great emphasis that is placed on the role of behavioural experiments. These planned searches for new, personal, direct evidence can be critical in facilitating the patient's fresh interpretation of the significance of their intrusive thoughts.

It is advisable to tape the sessions and ask the patient to review the recording before attending the next session. It is advisable to provide concentrated treatment early on, say twice a week, and then gradually taper off to, say, one session every three weeks.

The sessions can be intense, busy, and demanding, and it is unreasonable to expect the patient to absorb and fully recall everything that has taken place. A review of the tape is particularly helpful when a session has been 'busy' and/or extremely emotional. One patient remarked, 'Listening to the tape really helped as we talked about so much, I had missed some things. It also helped me to come to terms with some issues or got me thinking about some of the things we discussed.' Some patients get so anxious during sessions that their recall is adversely affected, and here the tape is an aid.

Educational components

The assessments will reveal the patient's knowledge and appraisal of their intrusive thoughts, the specific content of their obsessions, their critical misinterpretations, and the consequences of the misinterpretations.

Armed with the information collected by and from the patient, the therapist introduces the educational component of the treatment, which begins with a description of the nature of obsessions, both normal and abnormal, giving particular attention to the fact that obsessions are fundamentally unwanted intrusive thoughts of an unacceptable character, and that almost everyone experiences them from time to time (Rachman and de Silva 1978; Salkovskis and Harrison 1984; Niler and Beck 1989; de Silva and Rachman 1997). It should also be pointed out that the content of normal and of clinically significant obsessions, those that are abnormally intense or frequent or distressing, are not noticeably different. The therapist emphasizes the universality of the phenomenon and encourages the patient to speak openly and freely about his/her experiences, in recognition of the fact that intrusive thoughts are a common experience and need not be kept secret. Experiencing obsessions does not indicate that the person is undergoing a unique experience, or is a freak because of the experience. The patient should be encouraged to describe some of their unwanted intrusive thoughts that are of little trouble and easily dismissed.

Discuss with the patient the two printed lists of common obsessions in List of unwanted intrusive thoughts (a) and (b) (Toolkit form 8), including those reported by people without a clinically significant problem, and give the patient a copy. The items on the list were collected from patients with obsessions, patients with other psychological problems, and people without significant psychological problems.

Most patients are surprised to learn that unwanted intrusive thoughts are reported by the overwhelming majority of people. Some patients are disbelieving and a few are dismissive, but the commonest response is relief. They are relieved to discover that they are not weird, not freaks of nature, not outsiders. The knowledge that almost everyone has comparable thoughts is an important step towards normalizing their experiences and their self-concepts.

A 22-year-old woman was tormented by recurrent intrusive sexual thoughts, which could be set off by the sight of any attractive young man. She often imagined herself engaged in vigorous and even violent sexual acts with them. As she was extremely religious, had strict views on appropriate sexual behaviour, and was about to get married to an equally religious young man, these thoughts were utterly repugnant and unacceptable to her. At first she reacted to the didactic information with disbelief and horror, but gradually came to accept it. When she was able to discuss her intrusive thoughts with her fiancé, she was relieved to learn that he accepted the information without hesitation and he revealed to her that he too experienced unwanted intrusive thoughts. After a slow start she responded well to 10 sessions of cognitive behaviour therapy.

The second part of the educational component consists of a description of the treatment model, namely that unwanted intrusive thoughts become clinically significant, obsessional, if and when the person interprets them as being of great personal significance. Examples of unwanted intrusive thoughts that are regarded as being trivial, and others that often are regarded as being of great personal significance, should be provided, supplemented by examples that are elicited from the patient him/herself. Patients are provided with a brief rationale of the treatment plus references (see An explanation of the treatment: Toolkit form 9).

Most drivers get angry on occasions, and even curse under their breath or openly (e.g. 'I will kill you'). However, they seldom take seriously the aggressive feelings they experience while at the wheel; they soon calm down and dismiss their aggressive reactions as unimportant. In contrast, if a driver has a fleeting idea of deliberately running down a pedestrian, for no reason, that can cause problems. If the driver interprets the idea as showing that they harbour homicidal wishes, it becomes very upsetting. Do you ever have silly thoughts while driving? Or at other times? Do you ever have silly, unwanted thoughts about religion, or sex, or aggression? If so, which of these silly thoughts bother you and which do not? Do you know why some thoughts bother you and others do not?

Here it can be helpful to discuss the particular content of the patient's main obsessions. It is explained that there are three common themes in obsessions: aggression (harm), blasphemy, and unnatural/unacceptable sexual themes or urges (e.g. molesting, or doubts about sexual identity). After establishing the category into which the patient's obsessions fall, ask why the other themes do not feature in their obsessions. Generally, this leads the patients to recognize that the contents of their obsessions are closely connected to their values— they 'catastrophize' about thoughts/images that bear on their keenest values—and not about 'insignificant' images/thoughts.

It is then explained that as the personal significance attached to the unwanted thoughts increases, so the frequency and distressing quality of the experience both increase. Likewise, when the personal significance attached to an unwanted intrusive thought is lowered, there will be a decrease in the distress and frequency of the obsessions. The therapist then explains why unwanted intrusive thoughts arise in the first place, including descriptions of how stress or anxiety can give rise to a significant increase in the frequency of such unwanted thoughts.

> Unwanted thoughts can cause distress and it is quite natural for people to resist them, to fight them off. However, trying to suppress these intrusive thoughts can unfortunately cause them to increase! The harder you try, the worse they become.

In the next part of the educational component, the therapist explains the nature of neutralizing activities, both mental and overt, and how they can have an adverse effect on the obsessional experience. Neutralizing refers to any attempt made to 'put right', correct, change, or cancel the obsession. Common examples include: a compulsive act that counters the thought, generally in order to protect someone from harm; denying the thought; fighting it; saying a protective prayer or phrase; visually re-animating the victim/s; bringing them 'back to life'; and so on. Much neutralizing takes place internally (mentally) and can require intense concentration, leading to exhaustion. The main forms of external neutralization are compulsive checking, cleaning, and ordering. In the short term, these attempts at neutralization are often successful in reducing a certain amount of anxiety/discomfort, and these effects are typically achieved quite promptly. In the longer term, however, acts of neutralization serve to protect the idea that the thoughts are indeed of great personal significance and that the distress or the feared event might well have occurred if the patient had failed to carry out the neutralizing act. In fact, the distress, which arises from an unwanted intrusive thought, will diminish spontaneously, albeit a little more slowly than occurs after a deliberate act of neutralization.

In other words, the patient's belief that the distress would have continued except for the fact that he/she carried out a counter, neutralizing act, is incorrect. When appropriate, this point can be illustrated by another demonstration in which the person is asked deliberately to form one of his/her less disturbing obsessions, and on one occasion follow it by a deliberately neutralizing act, and on a second occasion to refrain from neutralizing. In this way, the patient is able to discover that the distress occasioned by his obsession will diminish spontaneously, and that it is not necessary to neutralize it. Where appropriate, the demonstration can then be repeated with a more disturbing obsession to consolidate the point. In tackling these beliefs, behavioural experiments can be extremely helpful.

Demonstration

Ask the patient to form a selected obsession; record the distress it produces and the urge to put it right, to correct it. Under condition (a) ask the patient to correct it (neutralize it), record distress and urges. Under condition (b) form the obsession but refrain from correcting it. Record distress and urges immediately and again 10 min later.

Attention is then turned to the effects of persistent avoidance behaviour (e.g. avoidance of sharp objects, school playgrounds, churches, and so on). Here too, the immediate effect of executing escape or avoidance behaviour is to achieve a degree of relief from anxiety in the short term, but in the long term the troublesome beliefs are protected from extinction. For example, 'If I had not taken care to avoid the children's playground, I certainly would have experienced the aggressive thoughts and might have lost control and acted on them'.

The occurrence of unwanted intrusive thoughts, particularly those of a morally repugnant character, can give rise to shame and embarrassment, and as a result are concealed, often for decades. As with the earlier examples, it is explained that concealment protects the person from shame and embarrassment but has the longer-term effect of passively confirming the exaggerated significance that has been attached to the obsession. Concealment also inadvertently protects the catastrophic misinterpretations because the person is not exposed to the views of other people or to evidence that might disconfirm the interpretation. The person may be extremely reluctant to seek treatment, or even comfort, because it would involve disclosure of what they believe to be shameful, morally repugnant ideas. (The psychometric assessments and clinical interview can be incidentally therapeutic for people with concealment, 'How did they know to ask me the questions? I can't be the only one with these thoughts'.)

The patient is then told about the occurrence of the cognitive biases, and in particular, thought–action fusion. They are told that vulnerable people can interpret an intrusive unwanted thought as increasing the probability of the feared event occurring and/or feeling that having had the thought or image is morally equivalent to carrying out the repugnant action. It is also explained that the concealment of these cognitive biases ensures their continuance.

The concept of inflated responsibility and its role in obsessive-compulsive disorder (OCD) is explained, plus the need to take steps to deflate any exaggerated tendencies the patient may experience. The last part of the educational component consists of information pertaining to the relationship between depressive mood and OCD, and depression and obsessions in particular. Namely, that there is a close association between obsession and depression but the sequence in which the two phenomena affect each other can vary. Often the obsessions cause a depressive mood but in other instances, a depressive mood is followed by an increase in obsessional activity.

Many patients will have had medication prescribed for their problem and it is necessary to elicit from them what their experiences have been with the medication, including side-effects, withdrawal effects, and, importantly, how the patient interprets the obsessions in the light of their reaction to medication. The provision of cognitive treatment can proceed in the usual manner for patients who are taking medication. In cases with significant depression, the provision of anti-depressant medications can facilitate the psychological treatment.

Some patients find the analogy of radio noise useful in appraising their unwanted intrusive thoughts. These thoughts can be regarded as the noise and not the signal—they are not significant. The true signals, that is the person's true values and beliefs, are what count and not the irrelevant noise. Here the therapist demonstrates by fiddling with the radio, distinguishing between the noise, which is off-station, and the true signals.

Demonstration of the difference between noise and signals

The educational steps are supplemented with printed material described earlier (see Toolkit forms 8 and 9). Before proceeding to the second stage of treatment, ask the patient to explain the treatment model in their own words, as this will reduce the likelihood of misunderstandings or confusion. Make a written record of the patient's explanation.

CHAPTER 5

Treatment—stage 2

After completion of the educational component, the therapist explains what he/she and the patient will each be expected to contribute to its success. The therapist explains that the purpose of treatment is to help the patient replace the catastrophic misinterpretations with more realistic and benign explanations of their intrusive thoughts, and to supplement these therapeutic attempts with deliberate and persistent modifications of the associated behaviour (i.e. reduction of avoidance, neutralization, suppression, concealment). It is also explained that the patient has the most active part in the treatment, both in the collection of data and in the close examination of the interpretations of obsessions, plus their intrepid attempts to refrain from carrying out the powerful urges to neutralize, suppress, and avoid. As with the educational component, the description of the treatment aims and procedures is supplemented with written material (see An explanation of the treatment: Toolkit form 9).

The patient is told that a typical course of treatment requires between 8 and 12 one-hour weekly sessions. Booster sessions are planned as necessary, and review and follow-up meetings are always arranged. It is explained that much of the treatment process involves 'homework exercises' and that the processes are directed and instigated during treatment sessions, but that between-session events are crucial.

As an aid to the therapist, a Session-by-session progress chart sets out the structure for each session (see Toolkit form 6). At various stages in the progress of treatment, certain agenda items are of central interest (e.g. an emphasis on specific behavioural experiments) and other items not relevant (e.g. the survey may have been completed at an earlier stage of treatment). Hence, the therapist should use the Session-by-session progress chart flexibly, modifying it as needed during the full course of treatment.

Reduction of significance

The aim of this part of the treatment is to identify the specific obsessions and any associated abnormal behaviour, to help the patient overcome the catastrophic misinterpretations of their obsessional experiences, and to promote the substitution of a benign alternative.

The expectation is that, to the extent that the therapist and patient succeed in replacing the catastrophic misinterpretation of the obsessional activity with a benign alternative, the frequency and intensity of the obsessions will be diminished or even disappear. The direct cognitive treatment is supplemented by behavioural change techniques to deal with unwanted avoidance or neutralization, and again, it is expected that success in dealing with the problem behaviour should be followed by a reduction in the frequency and intensity of the obsessions.

The major components of the treatment are:

1 assessment of the nature and personal meaning the person is attaching to his/her obsessions;
2 attempts to promote the elimination of the catastrophic misinterpretations and their satisfactory replacement;
3 supplementation by attempts to modify the associated abnormal behaviour, avoiding avoidance, refraining from thought suppression, and neutralization.

A great deal of attention is given to the patient's interpretation of the meaning and significance of these obsessions, and to the meaning and significance of the frequent occurrence of the obsessions. A detailed account of any escape and avoidance behaviour should be obtained, plus any information about thought suppression, neutralizing activities, and attempts at concealment.

The patient should complete the Personal significance scale (see Toolkit form 2), with the therapist's assistance (items 5, 7, 12, and 15 are buffer items, and can be ignored by the therapist).

There are essentially three ways to collect all this information:

1 by detailed clinical interviewing;
2 the use of psychometric measures (especially the Personal significance scale);
3 the data collected by the patient in regular between-session reports.

An attempt is made to find out which methods the patient is using at the present time to deal with their obsessions and how effective each method is. It is also worthwhile finding out which methods have been tried in the middle and distant past, and with what effects. This information can be valuable in formulating the details of the treatment programme—plainly one does not want to recommend tactics or procedures that have been found to be ineffective. It is presumed here that self-discovered methods that are effective are consistent with the present theory, i.e. that they involve corrective interpretations of the significance of the thoughts. Self-discovered methods that leave the putative misinterpretations of the significance of the obsessions unchanged are of little value.

Before embarking on the reappraisal of the significance of the intrusive and unwanted thoughts, a full analysis is advisable. This covers the patient's spontaneous interpretations, strength of belief, evidence and reasons for the interpretation, contrary evidence and reasons, spontaneous methods of resisting the thoughts and their efficacy, effects of formal treatment, and so forth.

A sample work sheet that covers these aspects of the significance given to the thoughts is shown in Toolkit form 3(a): Unwanted intrusive thoughts.

Toolkit form 3(a): Unwanted intrusive thoughts
Work sheet

Date: Participant:

The significance of unwanted intrusions

(Therapists: use a fresh sheet for each important unwanted intrusive thought)

1. Statement of most important unwanted intrusive thoughts (UITs), as described by the patient, in the patient's own words.
    (a)   *e.g. I wish to have sex with a religious figure*
    (b)   *e.g. am I a hypocrite?*

2. A statement of the significance that the patient attaches to the UIT, in the patient's own words.
    (a)   *e.g. it means I am sinful and will go to hell*
    (b)   *e.g. I can't be a sincere believer*

3. Ask patients to rate how strongly they believe in the interpretations (significance) they attach to the UIT, on a scale from 0 (not at all) to 100 (totally certain that this is correct).
    UIT 1: (a)   *e.g. 80%*   (b)   *e.g. 55%*   (c)
    (i)   What are the reasons for this interpretation?
           e.g. only a terrible sinner would have such disgusting thoughts
    (ii)   What are the reasons against it?
           e.g. I don't really wish it
    (iii) What important evidence is missing?
           e.g. can't say

(iv) How can you collect it? (surveys, behaviour, exposure, etc.)

e.g. don't know

3. Can you think of some alternative explanations?

e.g. no

4. What would your close friends/relatives think of your interpretations of your thoughts? (details—who, when, etc.)

e.g. they would be shocked

5. How do they interpret your reported thoughts?

e.g. can't say

6. If a very close friend of yours reported similar thoughts, what would you think of him/her?

e.g. I'd pray for them

7. How would you interpret his/her thoughts?

e.g. a sad problem for them

8. If a close friend asked you for advice about how to deal with his/her unwanted thoughts, what would you recommend?

e.g. pray? get medical help?

9. Why do you conceal your thoughts, if you do?

e.g. they are disgusting

10. Does this concealment work (help you, harm you)?

e.g. neither

10a. What exactly will happen if you cease to conceal your thoughts?

e.g. people will reject me

11. Why do you avoid places/people?

e.g. church—because I might have the thoughts there

12. Does it work?

e.g. yes

    12a. What exactly will happen if you cease to avoid?
    e.g. bad thoughts

13. What methods do you use to prevent the thoughts?
    e.g. block them, pray?

14. Do they work?

e.g. no

    14a. What exactly will happen if you stop preventing the thoughts?
    e.g. can't say

15. What methods do you use to get rid of the thoughts?
    e.g. pray

16. Do they work?
    e.g. not usually

    16a. What exactly will happen if you stop trying to get rid of the thoughts?
    e.g. nothing

17. How many of your methods of trying to avoid, prevent or remove your unwanted intrusive thoughts have failed?
    e.g. all

    17a. Why did each of these fail? (in participant's own words)

        [Therapist: now go on to: (a) Alternative explanations (Toolkit form 11); (b) The reactions of friends Toolkit form 15) (when these two steps are appropriate).]

After completing this detailed appraisal of the significance, proceed to an analysis of the evidence for and against the significance, and the reasons for and against the significance.

Specific cognitive tactics

Here the aim is to grasp the content of the thoughts and their significance for the patient, plus the evidence for and against the patient's interpretation of the significance of the thoughts. The best, strongest, and most persuasive evidence consists of the patient's own experiences—hence the critical importance of behavioural experiments, monitoring the effects of inhibiting the urge to neutralize, and so on.

Evidence

Ask the patient to list the reasons for his/her interpretation of the significance of the intrusive thoughts (the significance is garnered in the initial interview by Toolkit forms 2 and 3).

1 The thought (image, impulse) . . .
2 It means that . . .
3 Reasons for . . .
4 Reasons against . . .

Missing evidence

Can this be obtained by personal mini-surveys, exposure exercises, reading, behavioural experiments? (See below.) For example, will the church really reject a patient who is struggling against obviously abnormal blasphemous thoughts?

Examples

Some of the reasons advanced by patients:

◆ Normal people don't have such weird thoughts.
◆ These thoughts mean that I am abnormal.
◆ Whenever I am with elderly people/children, I feel anxious and that proves that I am weird and cannot be trusted.
◆ The bodily sensations that I sometimes experience while having the intrusive thoughts mean that I really have repugnant sexual/aggressive wishes.
◆ I sometimes have dreams of carrying out unacceptable sexual acts and that means I really wish to do so.

- One day I will lose control and carry out the unnatural acts.
- I sometimes have images of carrying out aggressive acts and that means that I really wish to do so.
- Perhaps I am going crazy.
- I have repeated images of engaging in unacceptable sexual practices and that means I am really weird.
- If these thoughts continue, I will end up crazy.
- I get so upset by these thoughts that they must be significant, important.

Patients should be encouraged to describe all of their reasons for attaching great personal significance to the intrusive thoughts, and then asked to talk about the evidence to support these reasons and evidence that goes against the reasons.

The work sheet Cognitive tactics (Toolkit form 10) will assist in collecting, collating, and testing the evidence and reasons for the patient's interpretation. A sample with illustrative answers is shown in Toolkit form 10(a).

Toolkit form 10(a): Cognitive tactics

This thought (or image or impulse) means that:

e.g. I am sinful, disgusting, immoral

My reasons for believing that meaning are as follows:

e.g. I should be holy and respectful to this religious figure

The specific evidence for believing that meaning is:

e.g. I often have the thought and it is worse in church

The reasons for disbelieving that it really means that include the following:

e.g. I don't really want it, I love and revere this figure

The specific evidence for disbelieving that it really means that includes:

e.g. can't say

What do other people who know about your thoughts, e.g. friends or relatives, think they mean?

e.g. no one else knows

Do you know their reasons for thinking so?

e.g. N/A

If you do not have the information from them, are you willing to ask specific people?

e.g. maybe

These general enquiries are supplemented by specific questions, along the following lines:

- How many times have you had these intrusive, unacceptable/aggressive/sexual/blasphemous thoughts?
- How many times have these intrusive thoughts been followed by acts of aggression (to children, the elderly, etc.), or embarrassment (e.g. shouting obscenities)?
- Or been followed by unacceptable sexual acts?
- Or been followed by sacrilegious acts?
- How many times have you experienced these disturbing sexual/anxious sensations?
- How many times have these sensations been followed by unacceptable acts of aggression/sex?
- How many times have your disturbing images been followed by carrying out the act?
- Have you ever had disturbing dreams about yourself behaving unacceptably or disturbingly badly?
- If so, were the dreams followed by the unacceptable acts you dreamed about?
- Has any doctor said that you are in danger of ending up crazy?

The case of a 43-year-old practising Catholic illustrates several features of religious obsessions. As a child he was given a bible that contained a disturbing picture of the devil. Shortly after he began experiencing intrusive images and thoughts about the devil, and he tried to neutralize them by praying and repeating the statement, 'I love God and God alone'.

During treatment he made the connection between his religious obsessions and his harm obsessions, leading to a reinterpretation of his 'blasphemy' as one manifestation of a psychological disorder, obsessive-compulsive disorder (OCD). He made good progress and reported decreasing frequency of the religious obsessions, noting that the distress and interference declined so much that he was able to read a book for the first time in months. We reviewed his progress and he reported a major shift in his beliefs about religious obsessions, and felt that God would not want him to suffer. He also concluded that there is no evidence that his obsessions 'repel God'. We reviewed the adaptive implications of changing the meaning of his religious obsessions, and then spent the remainder of the session introducing the ideas of moral and probability thought–action fusion. He felt that this played a role in his reluctance to challenge his harm obsessions, and agreed to begin to challenge the negative meaning placed upon ambiguous events or coincidences. His Personal significance scale scores for religious obsessions showed a large decrease (especially in the need to block or neutralize). The items covering harm obsessions showed small reductions but little change in the need to block or neutralize these obsessions.

Ideas of hell and the Devil have a way of cropping up in religious obsessions and at times the distinction between religious and personal interpretations can be blurred. In these cases, advice given to the patient by a religious authority or counsellor can be helpful, provided that the therapist has the patient's permission to let the authority know of the OCD problem in advance. Almost invariably, the religious adviser provides clarification and comfort, and supports the psychological therapy.

Reasoning about religious obsessions is also helped by elucidating the exacerbating effects of low mood, and by the patient's continued acceptance by the religious adviser and other members of the congregation.

The next case excerpt illustrates the analysis of alternatives to a harshly negative self-interpretation of a patient's religious ideas. A devoutly religious 26-year-old engineer sought help for his persistently troubling obsessional ruminations about whether or not he was worthy of his religion; they were preoccupying, distressing, and partly disabling. He had become asocial and had given up his Sunday-school teaching because he felt that he was a sinner and a religious hypocrite, unworthy of the responsibility. The ruminations were triggered mainly by his recurrent intrusive sexual images and thoughts, which he regarded as sinful abominations. As a hopeless hypocrite, he was no longer fit to teach young people. His religious counsellor was helpful but the obsessions persisted.

Patient: My religious doubts are so intense, and they are especially bad just when I need to rest.

Therapist: Can you explain?

Patient: They are worst when I get home tired after a full day at work. I am so shallow, a hypocrite.

Therapist: So, they are worse when you are tired?

Patient: Yes, definitely.

Therapist: And how about when you are feeling low?

Patient: Oh yes, then they become unbearable.

Therapist: So it seems that your religious doubts get worse when you are tired or low. Is that correct?

Patient: Yes.

Therapist: Do you remember if you ever had the unwanted sexual images two years ago and more, before your episode of depression?

Patient: Yes, I've had them, on and off, since I was about 16.

Therapist: What do you make of the fact that prior to the depression the images didn't make you feel like a religious hypocrite?

Patient: I can't say. Maybe the depression helped to make me feel hypocritical. I was feeling so low and pretty worthless.

Therapist: At least three factors seem to contribute to your intense self-doubt and religious ruminations—tiredness, low spirits and depressing self-criticism.

Patient: So it seems.

Therapist: In general do you think that important religious and philosophical matters are influenced by tiredness and low mood?

Patient: No, not really. The issues are deeper than that. They transcend tiredness and mood.

Therapist: Could it be that your unceasing ruminations, self-examinations, and self-doubting are more influenced by your psychological mood and tiredness than by transcendental issues?

Patient: It seems possible.

This excerpt illustrates the opening of a fresh alternative explanation of the patient's religious ruminations by eliciting psychological factors that may contribute to the person's ruminations.

The following case history illustrates how the cognitive tactics are used to prepare the way for behavioural experiments. A 21-year-old mechanic was tortured by fearful thoughts that he might sexually assault children. His sexual experience was rather limited, largely because of his shyness and elevated moral standards. Nevertheless, he had surges of strong sexual feelings and these sometimes occurred in the apparent absence of any identifiable stimulus, leaving him baffled and troubled. When they occurred in the presence of children he interpreted them to mean that he was a potential predator. He was deeply troubled by these thoughts and, of course, avoided being alone with children.

We spent several sessions discussing his thoughts and experiences as a preliminary to setting up behavioural experiments and planned exposures. Early on he was asked if he knew any sexual predators. He did not. All of his information on the subject was derived from newspaper and TV reports and these had left him with the idea that all of a sudden, out of the blue, and without warning, the predator loses control of himself and carries out his horrible activities in a crazed, trance-like state. It was explained that sexual predators typically carry out planned, deliberate acts to gratify themselves, and that mostly they had histories of very poor human relationships. The assaults are not the result of a sudden and inexplicable breakdown in which the person runs out of control, trance-like. He was given recommended reading to inform his view of predation.

He had never behaved in a sexually inappropriate manner, with adults or children. He was a popular and respected member of his large, extended family, and was given many responsibilities. He was trusted.

We then examined the effects of his attempts to gain some peace from his awfully disturbing thoughts. The persistence of the thoughts was evidence of the futility of his avoidance behaviour, of his endless internal debates, of his mental neutralizing. It was not working. An alternative was needed and he was introduced to cognitive theory and therapy.

He originally justified these types of safety behaviour as necessary to prevent a breakdown and a catastrophic loss of control. He felt that he was potentially dangerous and could not risk being in the presence of children. Specifically, he predicted that he would get anxious and may even molest a child. After suitable planning he engaged in a series of graded behavioural experiments in order to collect information about his feelings and his behaviour in the presence of children, starting with a snack at the local Macdonalds. His dire predictions were disconfirmed in test after test. As predicted, he did experience anxiety, in decreasing amounts, but there was no hint, not even the merest whisper, of inappropriate behaviour. He did not lose control, he did not break down, he did not enter a trance.

All of this accumulating information was progressively absorbed, and slowly but surely his personal significance ratings declined. The treatment, comprising 23 sessions, was effective.

Fear of loss of control

Many patients, especially those who suffer from recurrent intrusive impulses, fear that one day they will lose control and carry out some horrible catastrophic act. As a result, they strain under an intense self-imposed need to exert iron control and self-discipline, each day. They tend to monitor and over-monitor all of their thoughts. They are constantly on guard, and feel it is essential to be so.

The reply to the question of why they have never carried out their recurrent dreaded obsessional thoughts can take several forms:

- I would have done so but for the fact that I was careful, vigilant, and self-disciplined.
- but I fear that one day I will lose that control.
- I will become so anxious that I lose control.
- I will feel so anxious and out of touch that I will lose control.

- I will be so drugged by medication that I will become confused and lose control.
- I will carry out the horrible action in my sleep.
- because I take care to lock up all the knives and sharp instruments.
- because I keep well away from children.
- because I avoid being alone with children.

B.L., a 30-year-old woman, suffered from severe and incapacitating harm obsessions for over 11 years. Every single day she had recurring thoughts and impulses to harm other people, by stabbing them, or pushing them under a bus, or hitting them over the head with a baseball bat, and on and on. Inevitably, she had become widely avoidant and unable to keep a job. She was living in subsidized housing and ate her meals at a charitable institution. In fact she had never harmed anyone during the 11 years, and we ascertained from her that she was regarded by her family and friends as a particularly gentle and considerate person.

She feared that she might lose control any day at any time, and was constantly vigilant of her thoughts and actions. The intrusive thoughts were interpreted as indicating that she was a highly dangerous and unpredictable person, indeed a potential serial killer. Having battled with these intrusions many thousands of times, we asked her to recall if she had ever carried out a harmful act, and, after a lengthy interval, she said that once she had given her cat some cornflakes to eat, nearly causing it to choke. That sort of 'cereal' killer!

On the broader matter of whether she was given to impulsive, unpredicted actions, the reply was negative. She was able to describe herself as a reasonably self-disciplined person.

After compiling a list of situations that she consistently avoided, we asked her to predict what would happen if she exposed herself to these very places. The behavioural experiments disconfirmed the specific predictions and steadily undermined the idea that she was in danger of losing control and causing serious harm to others.

One aspect of the fear of losing control of one's thoughts that is of potential therapeutic value, lies in the distinction between important and unimportant thoughts. The patient is asked to describe their beliefs pertaining to the strict control of thoughts, and they generally make a clear distinction between controlling what they regard as important thoughts and the unimportant ones. Notably, they feel little need to control the unimportant ones—and they can do so with ease. If they 'define' an intrusive thought as very important, they exaggerate the need to keep it under strict control and, paradoxically, they then struggle to control it. In these cases useful progress can be made by helping the person to reassess the significance of the thought and the consequent need to exert strict control.

Tactics

Many of the reasons that patients give to explain why they have never, in years, ever carried out the dreaded act, readily lend themselves to behavioural experiments (see Chapter 7 for further details). For example, 'If under specified circumstances you refrain from using your usual self-discipline, what happens?'. Other reasons advanced, such as sleep-walking, present a challenge to the therapist's creativity.

Over-vigilance

If the patient engages in excessive self-monitoring of thoughts and is endlessly vigilant in the attempt to block unacceptable thoughts, steps are needed. They report feeling on guard all the time. The self-defeating quality of incessant vigilance and monitoring is discussed and, in particular, whether the vigilance has ever succeeded in providing peace or even relief. Examples advanced by patients include:

- I have to be on guard all the time.
- I am constantly examining my thoughts.
- Bad things will happen if I don't control my thoughts.
- I will feel responsible (guilty, to blame) if a bad thing happens because I failed to control my thoughts.
- Failing to control my thoughts would mean that I am an inadequate/weak person.
- I will be punished if I don't control my thoughts.

Proceed to a behavioural experiment in which the patient predicts the effects of refraining from incessant monitoring and then actually refrains for an arranged period or place. Patients find the idea of an 'off-duty' period helpful here—they can even make themselves a simple badge to wear during such periods to remind themselves that they are indeed off-duty. Then draw to their attention the contrast (usually minimal) when they remove the badge and resume duty. Do disasters occur during the off-duty period? Are they truly safer, or even feel safer, when they go back on vigilance-duty? Were their specific predictions confirmed or not? Did they lose control? The analogy with air traffic controllers, who are extremely vigilant on duty and hence, need off-duty rest, helps patients to construe their intense over-vigilance in a more reasonable, less demanding manner. Like the air traffic controllers, they need time off from intense scanning.

A 35-year-old-man suffered from an inflated sense of responsibility, which focused on his need to protect the health and safety of all of his relatives and friends. As a result, he was constantly on the lookout for important information about health and safety, stored piles of articles and magazines, and promptly told his relatives/friends about information relevant to their safety. The need to protect them was exacerbated by his cognitive bias towards thought–action fusion; he worried that merely thinking about threats to their safety actually increased the risk that they might be harmed.

Demonstration

1 Ask the patient to 'go on-duty', to be on guard and examine the significance of every thought. They are asked to examine the significance of all of their thoughts for 5 min: 'Act like an air traffic controller on duty'.

2 Then ask, ' During this 5-minute period on-guard, did you feel safer? Did you feel relaxed? Did it require a lot of concentration? Was it tiring?'

3 Then ask the patient to go 'off-duty' for 5 min: they are not required to be on-guard, to be vigilant, or to do any monitoring of the significance of their thoughts. The air traffic controller is taking a break, a rest; 'You are off-duty'.

4 Then ask, 'Did you succeed in taking a break? Did you truly feel off-duty? If so, did anything bad occur while you were off-duty? Did you feel safe? Relaxed? Tired?'

If the demonstration goes well, it can be extended to longer periods, for example, one full day on-duty, followed by one full day off-duty. Thereafter the patient is encouraged to draw conclusions about the role of excessive vigilance, and to desist from prolonged, self-defeating vigilance.

A major, common conclusion reached by patients is that the constant vigilance is unnecessary. They function well without the vigilance, in fact even better. They experience some liberation, are less tense and tired, and are able to use their mental energy for more rewarding, constructive purposes.

Alternative significance

Teasdale (1999) has argued convincingly that the removal of a mistaken interpretation is not sufficient: cognitive therapists should strive to help the patient formulate an alternative, more accurate, acceptable interpretation.

1 Are there any alternative meanings you can attach to the thoughts?

2 List the alternatives, and reasons for and against the alternative interpretations (see Alternative significance: Toolkit form 11).

How to collect new information

1 Deliberately chosen exposure exercises, *e.g. am I safe with children?*

In planning specific exercises, it helps to prepare a simple written plan, along these lines:

(a) The exact fear/ thought is . . . (*e.g. I may molest a child*).

(b) I predict that if I spend 10 min (near children in), *e.g. the park*, then I will feel (0–100) anxious, *e.g. 90%.*

(c) The probability of (molesting a child) is (0–100) (*e.g. 80%*)

(d) Actual report:

   (i) time spent, *e.g. 15 min*

   (ii) amount of anxiety, *e.g. 70%*

   (iii) probability of action, *e.g. 0%*

(e) Conclusions, *e.g. I get anxious but don't feel that I will lose control*

2 Where appropriate, conduct personal mini-surveys on friends and relations. Ask them, for example, 'Do you ever have unwanted intrusive thoughts?'; 'Has your attitude towards me changed since I told you about my thoughts?'; or 'What do you do about your thoughts?'. These surveys should be carried out on more than one person.

3 Conduct behavioural experiments, for example, on one day try to suppress the thoughts and on the next day refrain from doing so; on one day convince yourself the thoughts are highly significant and revealing, and on the next day convince yourself that they are mere 'noise', spend time with children/elderly.

As with the exposure exercises, it is helpful to prepare a simple plan:

1 The exact purpose of this task is to find out for myself what actually happens (*e.g. what happens when I stop fighting to block the thoughts*)

2 I predict that . . . (*e.g. if I stop fighting them for one entire day*), this is what will happen . . .

3 Actual report. This is what happened . . .

4 My conclusions are . . .

5 The exact purpose of the second task is to find out what happens if . . . (*e.g. I try my hardest to fight the thoughts, to block them*)

6 I predict that . . . (*e.g. if fight them hard for one entire day*) this is what will happen . . .

7 My conclusions are . . .

8 An alternative interpretation of my intrusive thoughts is . . .

This is an example of an alternative interpretation:

I was so anxious that I might molest children that I never gave myself a chance. I just kept away. But I have always known that I am fond of children. That remains true. My problem is that the awful anxiety interfered and made me doubt myself. And I feel that children sensed my uneasiness and didn't bother with me. But the real problem is my anxiety, not my behaviour towards children. And I can deal with the anxiety. What I have found out is that the anxiety needn't prevent me being with children, and I'm getting my confidence up. I am becoming a favoured uncle. The problem is anxiety, not molesting.

This is an illustration of the type of conversation that takes place:

Therapist: Everyone has a constant flow of thoughts, some of them are important but many are minor or trivial. Are your thoughts about harming other people important or minor?

Patient: Well, they are important of course. Very important.

Therapist: And how do you decide that they are important? How do you know that?

Patient: Because they are so upsetting. They cause me great distress.

Therapist: Any other reasons?

Patient: Well, they are so frequent. I get them every day, many times a day. They must be important or why would I get them all the time?

Therapist: So, they are important because they upset you so much and because they are so frequent?

Patient: Yes.

Therapist: Are there any other possibilities?

Patient: What do you mean?

Therapist: For example, what if the connection between the importance of the thoughts and the distress is reversed? What if you start off by defining them as important—the thoughts are important. It might follow that the thoughts cause you distress because you regard them as important.

Patient: What exactly do you mean?

Therapist: Let's see. If you regard a thought as non-important, does it upset you? Cause you distress?

Patient: No . . .

Therapist: If you regard a thought, or impulse, as non-important, will it go away?

Patient: Yes.

Therapist: And stay away?

Patient: Maybe.

Therapist: So let us think about it differently and see where it gets us. You interpret the thoughts/impulses as if they are highly significant, important for you.

Patient: Yes.

Therapist: What follows?

Patient: Well, if it's important, and objectionable, it certainly will upset me.

Therapist: And it is the important thoughts that we dwell on. The lesser ones come and go.

Patient: Yes, I can see that. Perhaps it is the important and significant thoughts that are upsetting me. And that is also why they hang about— because they seem to be important. I mean, if I think that they are important then I am not likely to ignore them, am I?

In this excerpt, the therapist tries to assist the patient to consider an alternative explanation of the association between the significance of the thoughts and distress/frequency.

Analysing the reactions of friends and relatives

The reactions of friends and relatives are potentially important sources of alternative information and interpretation (see Concealment of obsessions: Toolkit form 15). Illustrative answers are given in Toolkit form 15(a).

Toolkit form 15(a): Concealment of obsessions

1. Have you told anyone about your thoughts? (details) *e.g. my best friend*

2. If yes, has the person/s changed their behaviour towards you since you told them? (details) *e.g. no not at all*

3. Do they show signs of fearing you? *e.g. no, never*

4. Do they trust you? *e.g. yes*

5. Do they avoid you? *e.g. no*

6. Do they avoid being seen in public with you? *e.g. no*

7. Do they now avoid being alone with you? *e.g. no, we live together*

8. Do they now prevent you from being alone with young children? e.g. *no*

9. Do they exclude you? *e.g. no*

10. Do they call you sinful/immoral/wicked? e.g. *never*

11. If their behaviour has not changed in these (or related) ways, can you say what significance they attach to those thoughts of yours? e.g. *he thinks they are silly*

12. How would you react if a friend/relation told you that they were having obsessions somewhat similar to yours:

Would you fear them? *e.g. no*

Would you distrust them? *e.g. not at all*

Would you avoid them? *e.g. never*

If not, why not?

Analysing the fate of past obsessions

The patient's own experiences with past obsessions, what provoked them, and especially what led to their decline, can be of considerable relevance and importance (see The fate of past obsessions: Toolkit form 12). Usually they can recall a past obsession that has been lost. Sometimes they can be helped to pinpoint the events or thoughts that led to the disappearance of the obsession, for example, 'As my religious interests declined the blasphemous thoughts faded away'. The case illustrated in Toolkit form 12(a) nicely shows up the connection between the personal importance attached to the intrusive thoughts and the fate of the obsessions.

Toolkit form 12(a): The fate of past obsessions

1. When you first experienced your obsessions what did you think they meant?

2. What did you conclude?

e.g. I thought I was going crazy or weird

3. What did you do about it, if anything?

   e.g. worried alone

4. Did it work, did it help you?

   e.g. no

5. Did you tell anyone else about it?

   e.g. no

   (a) If not, why not?

   e.g. ashamed, disgusted

   (b) If yes, whom?

   e.g. N/A

   (c) What did they say, or do?

   e.g. N/A

6. Have any of your obsessions become less frequent/intense, or even completely gone?

   (a) Which ones?

   e.g. yes, as a teenager I had horrible anti-religious thoughts

   (b) When?

   (c) Explain why each one decreased.

   e.g. they just went away

   (d) What do you conclude from their disappearance?

   e.g. they are not permanent, not really me

   (e) Why did they weaken/go and other obsessions persist?

   e.g. can't be sure

7. Were any of your past obsessions followed by unacceptable, catastrophic behaviour?

   (a) Violent acts?

   e.g. no

   (b) Unacceptable sexual acts?

   e.g. no

    (c) Obscene acts

        e.g. no

    (d) Shouting in public?

        e.g. no

    (e) Making a nasty scene in church, others?

        e.g. I feared it, but no

8. What exactly prevented you from carrying out any of these acts? (The patient's replies can provide incisive questions to be tackled in behavioural experiments.)

e.g. managed to distract myself

Past treatments

The patient's reaction to previous treatments, psychological or medication, can be revealing. Their explanation for the positive/negative/neutral effects of the treatment can also reveal a good deal about the significance they attach to their thoughts and give clues as to what sort of information or experiences may have an impact on the obsessions (see Obsessions and past treatments: Toolkit form 13). As a guide to this part of the treatment, an enquiry outline is shown inToolkit form 13(a).

Toolkit form 13(a): Obsessions and past treatments

1. Have you received psychological treatment?

e.g. yes

    (a) If so, what and when?

        e.g. counselling for 2 years;meditation for 6 months

    (b) Did it help or not?

        e.g. both helped a bit but neither solved it

    (c) Explain its effects on you

        e.g. it helped to talk about it, to bring it out; the meditation gave me peaceful breaks

2. Have you received psychiatric treatment?

    (a) If so, what and when?

        e.g. yes 10 years; medication of various sorts

(b) Did it help or not?

e.g. helped to dull the intensity of the thoughts

(c) Explain its effects on you

e.g. shifted my serotonin levels

3. Have you received any self-chosen/other treatment, including reading, self-help manuals etc.?

(a) If so, what and when?

e.g. reading

(b) Did it help or not?

e.g. yes, it made me feel a bit less weird, less bizarre

(c) Explain its effects on you

e.g. I felt better about myself, more like a member of the human race

Your obsessions and your moods

Recognition that the interpretation that a patient places on their intrusive thoughts can be strongly influenced—in a positive or negative direction—by their mood states, often helps to loosen the rigidity of their beliefs about the nature of their obsessions. The information about mood–thought interactions can also make a useful contribution to their understanding of the mood-dependent nature of most obsessions and help to account for the effects of mood-influencing medication. The therapist can use Toolkit form 14 (Obsessions and moods), which includes a useful behavioural experiment involving a direct contrast between the effects of two distinct interpretations of the intrusive thoughts; it has broad uses and can have a remarkable impact; it also gets straight to the critical role played by the patient's interpretation of their intrusive thoughts.

Responsibility

Many patients with obsessional disorders struggle with an inflated sense of responsibility (Salkovskis 1985, 1998). They feel that they are pivotally responsible for caring for others and for preventing harm coming to them. They feel that they are obliged to carry out protective, preventive actions (such as compulsive checking in order to prevent harm coming to other people; Rachman 1976, 2001). Frequently it becomes necessary to explore the range and depth of a person's responsibility, and to take steps to modify it, if possible. Because the elevated sense of responsibility imposes an oppressive burden, and drives compulsive urges to check and to avoid, the threat of additional or increased responsibility can promote intense anxiety. Therefore, it is common for affected people to go to lengths to avoid any additions to their existing responsibilities (e.g. refusing promotion to a more responsible job, delaying or refusing marriage, etc.). This sense of responsibility plays into the obsessions and is a particular problem when thought–action fusion occurs.

The sense of responsibility can be extensive and reach amazing levels. One patient spent long hours on his balcony vigilantly scanning the neighbourhood to ensure that everyone was safe. Another patient felt impelled to protect all living creatures, including insects. She went so far as to ask people, even strangers, to be careful to avoid treading on earthworms in a public park.

Describe the concept of inflated responsibility, the over-wide and excessive sense of personal responsibility, and, if it is present, discuss with the patient more realistic and acceptable limits. The patient is encouraged to list their main responsibilities and, separately, common examples of how they overstep them (see Responsibility appraisal: Toolkit form 16, p. 141).

Most of the illustrative answers in Toolkit form 16(a) are taken from replies given by a young mother who was assailed by thoughts and images of harm. She felt primary responsibility for guarding her parents, husband, baby, cousins, neighbours, and made between four and ten telephone calls each evening to ensure everyone's safety. She felt guilty if she left someone out of the evening roll-call. This routine was reminiscent of prayers for the safety of relatives/friends, carried to extremes. Her need to protect people was intensified by thought–action fusion; whenever she had an image of someone being assaulted or having an accident she felt guilty for having put them at elevated risk—thinking of a misfortune increases the probability that it will occur.

Toolkit form 16(a): Responsibility appraisal

1. Do you feel a special responsibility for making sure that friends and/or relatives are safe and protected?

   e.g. yes, it is up to me

2. Do you make very sure to check that they are safe and well?

   e.g. repeatedly, on the telephone

3. Do you frequently feel that if some misfortune occurs to one of your friends/relatives you will be responsible?

   e.g. most every day

4. Do you feel especially responsible for checking the safety of your home and everyone and everything in it, before you leave?

   e.g. yes it is my responsibility

5. Do you feel especially responsible for checking the safety of your home and everyone and everything in it, before go to bed at night?

   e.g. yes

6. On many occasions, do you feel especially responsible for ensuring that everyone has a good time?

   e.g. especially at parties, family gatherings

7. Do you feel guilty if you have not made *absolutely* sure that your family/friends are safe?

   e.g. definitely

8. Do you spend a great deal of time and effort thinking about the safety and well-being of your family and friends?

   e.g. yes, far too much for my own good

Discuss also the connection between responsibility and control, and the absence of responsibility where no control is available. Then discuss the feeling of responsibility for thoughts, especially as it occurs in thought–action fusion. Use specific examples of partial and shared responsibility drawn from the patient's life. In the case of the young mother described above, we constructed a list of her main responsibilities (for her baby, herself, husband), and the minimal ones pertaining to the the neighbours and acquaintances. She reshaped her responsibilities and the corresponding behaviour, and also shrank her bias towards thought–action fusion.

Behavioural experiments designed to help the patient learn the different mental and emotional experiences associated with a transfer of responsibility, temporary to start with, can have a large impact (see Chapter 7).

Cognitive biases

Many people who are troubled by obsessive-compulsive problems display particular biases in their thinking. The inflated sense of responsibility, which is common in OCD, is associated with these biases.

1 The biased belief that the probability of a feared event actually occurring is greatly increased if the person feels responsible for preventing the event. For example, 'If I am responsible for ensuring that our house is safe from

fire, then the probability of the house burning is increased; but if someone else is responsible for protecting the house from fire, then the probability of the house burning down is negligible.' The bias is expressed by the feeling that 'when I am responsible, things are sure to go wrong'.

2 The biased belief that responsibility for preventing harm is independent of one's degree of control over the feared event. For example, 'I have no control over the safety of my distant father's driving and feel highly responsible for ensuring that he is safe from any harmful motor accident'. This is the responsibility-without-control bias.

3 The asymmetric attribution of responsibility refers to the tendency for affected people to feel inflated responsibility for misfortunes or harm coming to other people, and to minimize their responsibility for fortunate events/achievements/actions. They easily feel blame, but discount praise.

4 The most researched cognitive bias in OCD is thought–action fusion, consisting of the probability bias and morality bias, both of which rest on the underlying belief that one's thoughts influence external events.

   (a) The probability bias is the skewed belief that one's (fearful, troubling) thoughts can influence external events, can make them more probable. For example, if I have the thought that my relatives will have a motor accident, the risk to them is increased because I had the thought.

   (b) Morality bias is the skewed belief that one's (repugnant, unacceptable) thoughts are morally equivalent to carrying out the implied act. For example, having an unwanted, nasty, violent sexual image is as morally offensive as carrying out the unacceptable action.

As might be expected, when people who are prone to these biases experience these troubling thoughts, they feel compelled to cancel or suppress the thoughts. The thought–action fusion scale (Toolkit form 7), which forms part of the assessment battery, provides a way of recognizing people who are prone to these biases.

The therapist begins by identifying the patient's biases and explaining how they work, drawing attention to their self-defeating effects. These cognitive biases add to an existing inflation of responsibility, increase feelings of guilt, and promote attempts at thought suppression and neutralization. Altogether, an undesirable mixture of problems and events.

The patient is encouraged to notice the occurrence and effects of their biases and to take corrective steps, mainly by combating the false conclusions that emerge from thought–action fusion and other biases.

CHAPTER 6

Dealing with self-defeating safety behaviour

Safety behaviour

When they feel threatened and upset, patients with obsessional problems do as we all do—they seek safety. The main forms of safety behaviour evoked by obsessions are as follows:

- avoidance and escape behaviour
- concealment
- thought suppression
- neutralization
- reassurance seeking

Some of the tactics they use are helpful, but much of the so-called safety behaviour purchases brief relief at the cost of sustaining the underlying maladaptive cognitions. For example, a person who is assailed by obsessive images of molesting children learns to avoid or escape from congregations of children. The escape brings some relief of anxiety but all too often reinforces the erroneous belief that he/she might have committed a repugnant act but for the timely escape.

Concealing the nature and especially the repugnant content of the obsessions from friends and relatives seemingly protects the patient from rejection or worse. However, the very act of concealment can sustain the obsession—because it ensures that the patient never hears the balanced, calm, and moderating views of trusted others. The fearsome beliefs and fearsome interpretations of the thoughts remain unchallenged and hence, persist.

The role and the effects of safety behaviour will crop up at various points of treatment, and this important fact should be emphasized whenever appropriate.

> Your safety behaviour has not worked for you. Despite using your thought suppression/blocking/concealment/neutralizing/reassurance seeking, you continue to be tormented by the obsessions. Your safety techniques don't really work for you—so let us consider some preferable alternatives.

With very few exceptions they serve to conserve the false maladaptive interpretations of the unwanted thoughts and hence, should be discouraged. Because the notion that safety behaviour—(escape, avoidance, concealment, suppression, neutralization) can be harmful, comes as a surprise to many patients, it may be necessary to carry out some simple demonstrations that enable the patient to experience the effects of these types of safety behaviour.

The main forms of safety behaviour, plus some strategies for reducing and eliminating this behaviour, are as follows.

Avoidance

Avoidance or escape are the most common reactions to fear, and of course there are objectively dangerous situations in which they are essential. However, when the fear/anxiety occurs in objectively safe conditions, or when the fear is excessive, the pattern of escape or avoidance is unnecessary or worse. A 'successful' escape from a falsely perceived danger can help to preserve the false belief in the danger. So with obsessions, the patient who fears that he might molest a child ensures that he avoids them and never learns that the fear is a false one.

The most effective way to reduce the false or exaggerated fears is the well-established method of repeated, graded, gradual, planned exposures to the situation that is feared and avoided. It seldom fails. To maximize their effects, a full discussion of the reason for and the details of the repeated exposures is advisable. The exercises must be planned, graded, and gradual. In some circumstances it is helpful to start with a therapeutic modelling exercise in which the therapist/aide models the desired behaviour a few times before the patient copies it. The amount of fear/anxiety experienced on each exposure trial is recorded on the customary 0–100 (maximum) scale, the fear thermometer. The planned exercises are self-correcting. The fear and associated avoidance should decline progressively and if they do not, it indicates the presence of an error or omission. The plan or specific instructions may be confused or misleading or the planned exercises too steep. The obvious corrections are then made.

Concealment

Concealment is an important feature of obsessions. As it is generally the product of feelings of shame and fear, an analysis of the person's concealment can be a pathway to the core of the obsession. *What* are they hiding and *why*? It can be extremely embarrassing, humiliating, and even painful for people to reveal the content of their obsessions. They tend to leak the details slowly, bit by bit, only when they feel secure in therapy. In some cases, the patient finds it easier to provide a written description of the obsession. Even here one can encounter problems; some patients feel that disclosure of the obsession weakens their power of control, or can even invalidate their 'magical' powers of control. Other patients resist disclosure because they feel responsible for protecting their relatives and friends, and worry that by revealing the obsessions they might jeopardize the safety of these other people.

Other anticipated consequences of disclosure that prevent the affected person from telling others of the content and frequency of the unwanted thoughts are shame and embarrassment. Even if they do not anticipate that people will recoil and then reject them for their obsessions, merely telling others about this repugnant private secret, will be upsetting because they feel so ashamed. Patients also feel that by telling others of their obsessions they will be revealing a hidden, unacceptable side of their personality. 'They will find out that I am weird, a freak'. 'It is so hard to talk about the thoughts as I feel defective and it is so humiliating'. Some patients are so concerned with embarrassment and shame that they agree to disclosure only if the therapist agrees to stop audiotaping, taking notes, or making any record of content of the obsession. In extreme instances of harm obsessions, some patients even fear that if they disclose the thoughts, it might lead to criminal charges or other legal consequences. Another reason advanced by patients who are reluctant to disclose the nature of the obsessions is that by making the disclosure they might thereby lose control of their thoughts. This can be particularly important for those patients who have a basic belief that it is essential for them to have total and constant control over their thoughts. For them, telling someone else or writing it out involves a potential loss of control. Somewhat related to this reason for inhibiting the disclosure of their thoughts is a 'magical belief' or cognitive bias that by saying out loud what the obsession is, or by writing it out, the patient will give the thought an added reality, thereby increasing the danger of losing ultimate control. For example, when attempting to disclose harm obsessions about her child, a mother said 'I don't want to say it out loud as it will attract negative energy and put my daughter in danger'. This phenomenon at times comes close to thought–action fusion (TAF) (Shafran et al. 1996; Rachman 1997c; Rachman and Shafran 1999).

The concealment of obsessions can add to the unfortunate consequences of obsessive-compulsive disorder (OCD). The concealment of the obsessions ensures that they will be preserved from disconfirming information provided by other people, and also preserved from the alternative explanations that other people might place on the significance of the thoughts. The distress caused by these horrific thoughts makes patients disinclined to mix with other people. A high proportion of the patients in our current sample had concurrent social anxiety. For example, patients who experience obsessions of causing harm to others, say young children or elderly people, avoid coming into contact with children or the elderly. Given that the content of many of the obsessions concerns the possibility of losing self-control and harming other people, it is understandable that people affected avoid social events in which they fear losing control. As a result, whatever social anxiety preceded the development of the obsessions, will be strengthened, and even if there was no pre-existing social anxiety, harm obsessions coupled with fear of loss of self-control can promote a fear of social occasions. Another unfortunate consequence of concealment is that it preserves the patient's view that the obsessions reveal their very worst qualities. Over time the patients develop idiosyncratic and isolated interpretations of their unwanted intrusive thoughts.

Concealment is considered to be a variant of avoidance behaviour, and to serve the same function. It provides short-term relief at best, but in the longer term helps to maintain the patient's catastrophic misinterpretations of their intrusive thoughts. Importantly, by concealing these obsessions from confidants, the patients preclude any chance of learning that trusted familiars place a significantly different and benign interpretation on the intrusive thoughts. Part of the reason for concealment is the patient's expectation, usually incorrect, that other people will place the same catastrophic interpretation on the obsessions.

These obstacles can be overcome with patience, and indeed the very process of disclosing the concealed material can reduce its inflated significance. Useful questions to encourage disclosure include:

- Have you kept these thoughts secret?
- Whom have you told? When and with what reaction ? Were they sympathetic or not?
- Are there particular people whom you would never tell? Why them?
- Did anyone react badly when you told them?
- When told of your obsessions did these people avoid you, shout at you, bug you, ignore it. . . . ?
- Did any of them change their attitudes and behaviour to you?
- If not, why not?

The aims of disclosure are to disconfirm the patient's expectations of the negative reactions of others and to change the significance attached to intrusive thoughts. By concealing their obsessions, patients cut themselves off from the moderating views of other people. No fresh air can enter the patient's closed, concealed universe of dread, doubt, and shame.

If a patient describes their intrusive thoughts readily and with pleasure, rather than reluctantly and with shame, embarrassment, and guilt, it is unlikely to be an obsession.

The disclosure to a friend or relative should be planned with care because an ill-conceived disclosure can backfire. The patient is encouraged to select trusted people who are sympathetic and psychologically minded, and may even need to practise with the therapist the type and amount of disclosure that is contemplated. As a safeguard it is best to plan and practise disclosures to more than a single person.

To assist in guiding the patient from concealment to disclosure, Toolkit form 15: Concealment of obsessions can be used.

Table 6.1 Concealment and disclosure: causes and consequences

Causes of concealment

People will recoil if they hear what my thoughts are

People will reject me if they know my secret thoughts

People will think I am crazy or dangerous if they know my secret thoughts

People will distrust me/fear me/avoid me if they know my secret thoughts

I will be ashamed/upset/guilty if I reveal the thoughts

I must strictly control the secret thoughts

If I lose control of my secret thoughts I might go crazy

If I lose control of my secret thoughts I might lose control of my actions

If I reveal my secret thoughts they could be used as evidence against me

If I reveal my secret thoughts people may contact the authorities

If I reveal my secret thoughts it will become 'official'; there will be a record

Revealing my secret thoughts may increase the probability of harm to others (probability TAF)

Saying the thoughts out loud is almost as bad, or as bad, as actually acting on the thoughts (moral TAF)

Patients' spontaneous tactics for controlling the thoughts (safety behaviour)

Neutralization

Thought substitution

Thought suppression

Avoidance of provocative stimuli/places (e.g. movies, playgrounds)

Internal debates/excessive rationalization/self-reassurance

Reassurance-seeking from others (without disclosure of thoughts)

Distraction

Self-medication (e.g. consuming alcohol)

Patients' reasons for disclosing

These thoughts make me feel bad/mad/dangerous

Need for reassurance

Attempt to shift responsibility

I cannot concentrate properly

It disturbs my life

It interferes with my personal relationships

I have to avoid so many places, people, etc.

I need to unburden

I need to obtain relief and liberation

Therapists' reasons for encouraging disclosure (to carefully selected, prepared people)

Patient needs fresh information

Patient needs fresh interpretation of the meaning of the thoughts

Promotes normalization of the experience of intrusive, unwanted thoughts

Promotes disconfirmation of anticipated rejection

Promotes disconfirmation of anticipated loss of control (mental or physical)

Promotes disconfirmation of anticipated harm to others

Promotes disconfirmation of anticipated TAF

Therapists' reasons for discouraging unselective, unprepared disclosures

Uninformed, unfamiliar people may strengthen a catastrophic interpretation of the meaning of the secret thoughts

It can cause unnecessary distress

It can lead to criticism, mistrust, and rejection

It can lead to increases in concealment

It can lead to increases in other safety behaviour

Source: Newth and Rachman 2001.

Overcoming the urge to suppress the thoughts — two techniques for cognitively reframing thoughts as meaningless noise

Many patients are understandably confused and troubled by the very fact that the obsessions are so frequent and keep coming back. 'They must be important, and even revealing because they are so frequent and so intrusive. Why do I keep having them?'

Therefore, when the therapist provides the educational component and introduces the idea that obsessions may be insignificant, mere noise in the system, it is not uncommon for patients to feel confused at first. 'If they are so insignificant, why do I keep having them?'

The explanation consists of two parts. First, we pay more attention to significant matters than to insignificant matters—hence, if the intrusive thoughts are regarded as *important*, then we pay more attention to them. If we regard the intrusive thoughts as unimportant, and many of our thoughts are unimportant, then we pay less attention to them. Secondly, it has been found that attempts to fight off, to suppress, unwanted, intrusive thoughts often produces the opposite result. They can become more frequent, not less frequent!

Demonstrations

Tell the patient, 'Your attempts to suppress your own obsessions haven't worked as well as you hoped. The obsessions keep coming back no matter how hard you try to block them. There are some simple, brief demonstrations that will show you the effects of trying to block the thoughts.'

1 When I tell you to begin, but not before, I want you to think about whatever you wish, anything at all. However, there is one exception—you are not to think about elephants! Whatever happens, block out, fight against any thoughts of elephants. It is forbidden to think of elephants.

Now, please close your eyes, relax, and think about anything at all, but NOT ELEPHANTS. Begin now.'

After 2 min, end the demonstration and ask for a report. In most instances the patients report some thoughts of elephants, sometimes indeed, entire herds.

2 For the second demonstration, ask the patient to provide one of their common but not too distressing obsessions, and repeat the exact instructions substituting the obsessional thought for elephants. That is, 'You can think of anything at all, but NOT the _____ (obsession). It is "forbidden" to think of the obsession.'

After 2 min, end the demonstration and collect the patient's report. They usually report experiencing the obsession for at least part of the time, despite their attempts at suppression.

3 This third, additional, demonstration is designed for patients who suffer from intrusive repetitive words, such as kill, hate, rape. The instructions are as for the earlier demonstrations but the relevant *word* is substituted for elephants.

The results of the demonstrations are discussed and provide a basis for recommending that the patient desists from trying to fight off, block, or suppress the obsessions. 'Let them simply float through your mind. Regard them as noise, just noise. Don't try to fight them off, or block them, or cancel them.'

Behavioural experiments to test the consequences of lack of suppression

Some patients feel that there is a moral need for them to fight off the thoughts, that if they cease fighting them, it means that they accept the thoughts. The therapist explains that there is no such moral imperative because the intrusive thoughts are not morally significant, or indeed significant in any way. Furthermore, moral or no, the attempts to fight off the thoughts do not work and have not worked for the patient.

Other patients believe that if they cease fighting off the thoughts something bad will happen and they will be responsible. They may believe that they are particularly responsible for protecting others and their attempts at suppressing thoughts are a necessary part of this protection—a form of safety behaviour. They may even feel that the dreaded misfortune (often vague and diffuse) has been prevented precisely because of their efforts at suppression.

In these instances, behavioural experiments are called for. Depending on the patient's beliefs, the experiments are directed at the inflated sense of responsibility and/or the belief that thought suppression makes people safer. As with all behavioural experiments, a simple plan is devised.

Behavioural experiment

1 The purpose of the experiment is to test whether or not . . . (e.g. other people are safer when I suppress the thought, than when I refrain from suppression).

2 I predict that when I suppress the thoughts for an entire day/week . . .

3 Report back.

4 The purpose of the opposite experiment is to test whether or not . . . (e.g. people are safe even when I totally refrain from thought suppression).

5 I predict that when I refrain from all suppression for one day/week . . .

6 Report back.

Discouraging neutralization

Closely related to suppression is neutralization. Suppression refers to attempts to block the obsessions and neutralization to cancelling out the effects of the obsessions. The therapist explains that obsessions frequently give rise to attempts to neutralize the effects of the thought; all too often these attempts at neutralization serve to confirm the mistaken importance that is attached to the obsession. Attempts at neutralization may make it more difficult to overcome the problem, and are therefore discouraged. Neutralization may take the form of attempting to substitute an acceptable thought, or trying to form a safely reassuring image in order to cancel out the unacceptable thought (e.g. reanimating a dead 'victim' by constructing an image of the person alive and active), or somehow to 'put matters right'. Neutralization can be internal, as in saying a corrective phrase or prayer, and it can be external, as in hand-washing.

As with hand-washing or compulsive checking, neutralizing generally provides prompt relief—but the relief rarely lasts. More neutralizing is needed. The trap is for patients to believe that the dreaded misfortune has been averted because they neutralized; this consolidates the fundamental misinterpretation of the significance of the intrusive thoughts.

It has been shown that the discomfort or dread that is reduced by neutralization has a natural tendency to decline even if the neutralizing act is omitted. It takes a little longer to go away but it does go. It is helpful for patients who go in for neutralization to experience this natural decline, and the following demonstration can be used. If the patient feels morally compelled to cancel out the obsession, to neutralize it, the demonstration should be complemented by an examination of the 'moral' component of the neutralization.

Demonstration

Select a clear and reproducible act of neutralization provided by the patient (e.g. blanketing the obsession with a counter-thought or a counter-image, saying a neutralizing phrase such as 'they are safe' or 'peace'). Ask the patient to form one of their obsessions, signal when they have it, hold it for 2 min or so, then carry out the neutralizing action. Did the formation of the obsession produce anxiety/discomfort? (0–100 scale). Was the neutralization action performed correctly? What effect did it have on the anxiety (0–100)?

Generally, the obsession will cause some discomfort, in the region of 30–40 on the 100 scale, but less than the discomfort that the patient's spontaneous obsessions produce. When the neutralizing act is completed the anxiety usually declines promptly, to say 10/100.

Then proceed to the second part of the demonstration in which the obsession is again formed, but this time the patient refrains from any neutralizing. If the obsessions provoked moderate anxiety (30–40), it will remain at about that level for a few minutes. Then engage the patient in a 10 min discussion of some unrelated subject, after which time, check the patient's level of obsession-anxiety again. Usually it will have spontaneously declined to 0 or close to that.

In this way the patient learns by experience that the anxiety and the urge to neutralize will decline without any special effort. Consequently, if they refrain from neutralizing, the anxiety will go away and of course, no great misfortunes will take place because they left their obsessions 'uncorrected'. If patients delay carrying out neutralizing for specified periods, such as 1, 5, or 10 h, they generally find that when the agreed time to neutralize finally arrives, they no longer feel the urge to do so (the delay tactic). When encouraging patients to delay neutralizing (or checking, etc.) it is best for them to set a specific period of delay (e.g. 4, 6, 8 h hence). Patients are also advised to refrain from carrying out internal debates about the validity of their obsessions. These debates are tiring, seldom resolved, and frustrating.

Behavioural experiments on the transfer of responsibility

Behavioural experiments can be most helpful in guiding the patient to an understanding of the heavy burden that inflated responsibility places on them (see Toolkit form 17: Behavioural experiment). A handy way of facilitating this recognition is by planning an experiment to measure the effects of a (temporary) transfer of responsibility to someone else, usually a spouse or parent. As a warm-up it can be helpful for the therapist to carry out a demonstration of the technique and effects of a transfer of responsibility during a session.

It is expected that the transfer of responsibility will result in a decline in over-vigilance and in tension, and also a reduction in any associated compulsive checking. The impact can be remarkable, as this case illustrates. A 35-year woman complained of an excessive fear of domestic disasters, especially of a fire destroying her home. She ruminated about her fears and of course, engaged in compulsive checking of the home. It took her up to 20 min to check and recheck the house before leaving it. By agreement with her husband a behavioural experiment was set up. It was planned that for six consecutive days they would compare the patient's emotional reactions on days when she retained her inflated sense of responsibility with days on which she transferred the responsibility to her husband. They alternated the days of responsibility and at the end of the experiment had collected data on three days when he was responsible and three days on which she was responsible. As predicted the patient found out that her self-imposed responsibility made her tense, moody, and ruminative. On the days when she transferred responsibility to her husband she felt liberated, relaxed, and better able to concentrate.

An illustration of the form of a suitable behavioural experiment on transfer is shown as Toolkit form 17(a), using this patient's responses.

Toolkit form 17(a): Behavioural experiment on transfer

1. The purpose of this experiment is to collect information about *the effects on me of a temporary transfer of responsibility.*

2. On . . . I will transfer responsibility to the following person/people . . .

   e.g. I will transfer responsibility for securing our home to my husband

3. I predict that I will (a) feel and (b) do the following. . . .

   e.g. I predict that I will feel terrible all day, worrying about the house and will be unable to concentrate at work

4. Report on the experiment
   (a) *On . . . we carried out the experiment at home.*
   (b) *I felt anxious on the first day and was very hesitant. Surpisingly I got used to it and then began to feel liberated. I did NOT ruminate about it and was able to concentrate just fine at work.*
   (c) *My predictions were not correct.*
   (d) *My belief that I could not do it was disconfirmed.*

Many patients with inflated responsibility find it extremely difficult to transfer responsibility, even for a few minutes. Sometimes one can find a simple and undemanding starting point, but the rigidity of the beliefs and feelings about responsibility cannot be overestimated, and the patient may be unwilling, or even unable, to risk any dilution of their self-imposed obligations. If the behavioural experiment approach fails to get off the ground, therapists should try other tactics. Often one searches around for the best way to get at the catastrophic interpretations, and what works wonderfully for one patient, may be a squib with another. Almost invariably one or several approaches will open the path to less catastrophic misinterpretations.

Dealing with self-doubt

Some patients are tormented by recurrent cycles of self-doubt:

- Am I a hypocrite?
- Do I truly love my husband?
- Am I attracted to people of my own gender?
- Am I a genuine believer?
- Am I morally flawed?
- Did I offend the priest six years ago?

In most instances the questions cannot be resolved and leave the person feeling drained, frustrated, and miserable. The attempts to find the answer are motivated by a belief that all such questions *must* be answered.

The patients is encouraged to substitute a more benign view, in which they assert or reassert the belief that they retain the power to select which questions to tackle and which ones to dismiss. 'I do not need to address that question and I will not.' The efficacy of this simple tactic can be strengthened by a behavioural experiment. The patient is asked to make a comparison between the effects of attempting to answer the question and the effects of the new tactic in which they assert to themselves that they need not address the question. In general, the experiment works well if the patient uses the alternative tactics for a full day at a time, and keeps a daily record of the frequency, duration, and intrusiveness of the self-doubting questions, and any associated distress. So for example:

Monday ('Try to answer the questions')
Frequency	= 5
Average duration	= 25 min
Degree of intrusiveness	= 7/10
Associated distress	= 45%

And on the following day:

Tuesday ('I do not need to answer this question')
Frequency	= 3
Average duration	= 1 min
Degree of intrusiveness	= 2/10
Associated distress	= 10%

Wednesday (revert to 'Try to answer the question' tactic)

Thursday (resume 'I do not need to answer this question')

After repeated contrasts of this type the person learns by direct experience that it is *not* necessary to make attempts to answer the questions and that gradually they observe a decline in the frequency and intrusiveness of the question(s). Importantly, they discover that refraining from needless self-debate is not followed by misfortune or distress.

Refraining from seeking reassurance

The repeated and often insistent seeking of reassurance about one's safety, or in the case of obsessions, the safety of others, is a form of maladaptive compulsive behaviour and is therefore discouraged. Friends and relatives are advised to withhold such reassurance—'It will interfere with your progress in treatment if I give that reassurance. It is against your interest.'

It helps patients to be informed authoritatively that the reassurance gives short-term relief but sustains the obsessions, and also to be reminded that they already *know* the reply to their request for reassurance. *They are not actually seeking information and nor will they receive any new information.* The reassurance-seeking is a maladaptive attempt to reduce anxiety and patients are urged to refrain from asking for such reassurance.

The use of pragmatic tests

Beck (1998, personal communication) has recommended using pragmatic tests to assist patients in overcoming their maladaptive beliefs and interpretations, and these tests can be very helpful in dealing with the maladaptive interpretations that fire the person's obsessions.

Beck asks the person whether they would be better off or worse off if they shed their maladaptive cognitions. Would your life be easier, more fulfilling, if you set aside these cognitions? Would your life be easier, more fulfilling if you substituted more accepting, realistic cognitions?

These questions are put to the patient, asking them whether their *specific* interpretations of the significance of their unwanted, intrusive thoughts are a help or a hindrance in their lives. 'Will your life be more peaceful if you can substitute an accepting, benign interpretation of these thoughts to replace your self-critical interpretations?' Construct with the patient two contrasting interpretations: one of their self-critical interpretations, and the other an accepting, benign interpretation. For example.

(a) These thoughts mean that I am a bad person, hypocritical, and possibly dangerous.

(b) These thoughts are mere noise. They tell me nothing of importance about myself. My behaviour and my principles are those I value and have chosen for myself. These thoughts are irrelevant.

Having constructed the opposing interpretations the patient is again asked whether they would be better off or worse off if they used interpretation A. The same question is then asked about interpretation B. 'Pragmatically, which interpretation is best for you?'

The interpretations are then used as the basis for a grand behavioural experiment. The patient is encouraged to adopt and endorse interpretation A or a full week, to convince themselves of its validity, and to record the effects of the interpretation on their feelings and behaviour, and on the frequency and intensity of their obsessions.

In the second week, they are encouraged to adopt and endorse, with conviction, the validity of the contrasting and benign interpretation B. As before, they record their feelings and behaviour during the week plus the frequency and intensity of the obsessions.

The aims of this behavioural experiment are to assess the pragmatic value of the two interpretations and importantly, to promote the patient's experience of life without the maladaptive interpretation of their intrusive thoughts. It can be liberating.

Patients who successfully adopt and endorse the contrasting interpretations for the period of the experiment often benefit remarkably. Success also strengthens for them the new, and welcome, explanation of their obsessions that the therapist has suggested.

If the patient has several obsessions, pragmatic behavioural experiments can be used to test each one in turn. In some cases, it is desirable to repeat the behavioural experiment for greater effect, and/or to extend the test period from 1 week to 2 or 4, or more, again for greater and more enduring effects.

CHAPTER 7

Tactics

Behavioural experiments

The behavioural experiments that play such an important part in treatment, are mini-experiments in which the patient tests the validity of specific expectations (e.g. my family will reject and avoid me if I tell them about my obsessions, if I attend church service I will lose control and shout obscenities, etc.). The patient's responses to the question, 'What exactly will happen if you (carry out the behaviour instead of avoiding, stop suppressing, etc.)'?, provides the best material for the behavioural experiments.

The purpose of the experiments is to allow the patient to collect direct, personal information pertaining to important obsessive-compulsive disorder (OCD) beliefs—and to do so in a thoughtful, planned manner rather than merely hoping for random events to occur. In order to facilitate an effective behavioural experiment, it should be planned with a specific stated purpose, and the simple procedure set out below can help. The experiments should be designed to collect information and in this way differ slightly from exposure exercises. Exposures certainly can uncover fresh information but this is incidental; in most instances the primary aim is to reduce fear. Behavioural experiments invariably have an exposure component but the primary aim is to collect information, information that bears directly on the belief under investigation. The experiments are particularly helpful when a patient is hesitant or sceptical about considering fresh interpretations and/or when they endorse more benign interpretations only in the clinic but not in the external situations.

There is a strong tendency for people to over-predict the likelihood and the unpleasantness of fear and other aversive events. The behavioural experiments also provide a simply and useful way of reducing such unwanted over-predictions. In some circumstances, it is desirable for the patient to be accompanied by a therapist/aide during the behavioural experiment.

The use of the Behavioural experiment form (Toolkit form 17) helps to structure the experiment, to make the purpose explicit and to encourage reaching a conclusion from the experiment. Illustrative answers are shown in Toolkit form 17(b).

Toolkit form 17(b): Behavioural experiment

1. The purpose of the experiment is to test the belief that ....

   e.g. I might inadvertently make someone pregnant by contamination

2. On _____ I will (go to, ask, tell, etc.) the following people/place.

   e.g. my female cousin's home

3. I predict that I will (a) feel and (b) do the following:

   e.g. (a) anxious (b) avoid using the bathroom

Report on actual event, a month later

1. On *e.g. Tuesday,* I carried out the experiment in/at: *e.g. my cousin's home*

2. I felt *e.g. slightly anxious,* and behaved *e.g. awkwardly.*

3. My predictions were correct/incorrect.

   e.g. partly correct but I was not nearly as anxious as expected

4. My belief that *e.g. I would contaminate her* was supported/disconfirmed.

   e.g. was not confirmed

It is very important to encourage the patient to carry out the behavioural experiences as soon as possible after the completion of the treatment sessions. The motivation to carry out the necessary work is highest at the end of the session but wanes if the patient postpones the implementation for several days.

The same advice to carry out 'homework exercises' sooner rather than later, when the patient's motivation is high, is applicable to all therapeutic manoeuvres, including mini-surveys, exposure tasks, and so on. As ever, the patient's direct experiences will carry greatest evidential value for them.

Carrying out mini-surveys

Just as patients over-interpret the significance and the meaning of their unwanted, intrusive thoughts, so they are inclined to assume that everyone else shares their catastrophic interpretations. For example,

If I think that my aggressive thoughts about children reveal the darker, danger-ous side of my character, then it follows automatically that everyone else will reach the same conclusion—if they knew about my thoughts they would reject me as a dangerous, evil person.

But do other people over-interpret the significance of one's obsessions? Is it true? Collect the evidence.

The aim of the mini-survey is to collect evidence about other people's thoughts and attitudes, from the people themselves, rather than allow the patient to infer or merely guess what other people think or are likely to think.

Ask the patient to select a few people whom they trust and whose opinion they value. It should be agreed in advance that at least a few people will be asked to provide their views; asking only one person can lead to a distorted conclusion. In most instances the mini-survey begins with a question or two about the respondent's own thoughts.

1 Do you ever have unwanted, intrusive thoughts or images?

If yes:

2 Do you think they are important; do they mean something important about you?

If so:

3 What? Why?
4 What do you do about them?
5 Have you told anyone else about these thoughts?
6 What did they say or do?
7 If I told you about some of my unwanted, intrusive thoughts would you be willing to listen?

If yes, go ahead, describe the thoughts and explain that you are trying to overcome them with the help of a psychologist.

Remember the reaction of each person and note whether their behaviour/atti-tude towards you changes after you have spoken to them. After completing a few such interviews, review the evidence and draw conclusions (Mini-survey: Toolkit form 18).

A memorable mini-survey was carried out by a patient who had obsession-al fears of harming his 7-year-old nephew. He was convinced that his (older) brother and sister-in-law would be horrified to hear of these fears and would ostracize him. Finally, one Sunday afternoon, he told them of his fears. The sister-in-law listened carefully and was sympathetic and reassuring, but his dismissive older brother showed little interest. Early in the evening, the brother and sister-in-law decided to go out for dinner and asked if the patient would agree to look after the child for a few hours while they went out. The patient was astonished, but after much hesitation he agreed to mind the child if they promised to return within two hours. They did and he cared for his nephew.

Later, the therapist asked the patient what his relations' request for child-minding told us about how they interpreted his obsessional fear. He concluded that, 'they don't take my nasty thoughts seriously'. This event and its meaning helped the patient to develop a more benign explanation of his intrusive unwanted thoughts.

Exposure without neutralization

The familiar exposure techniques can be of considerable value, even though the obsessional experiences are covert and seemingly inaccessible. If the person reports significant avoidance behaviour, this indicates the usefulness of carrying out exposure exercises. With preparation, by relaxation and/or modelling, the person is encouraged to enter those very situations that provoke the obsessional ideas (such as using knives in a relaxed natural manner, walking past school playgrounds if the obsessional thoughts centre on the possibility of aggressive acts towards children, etc.). Frequent repetition of these exposure exercises leads gradually to a decline in fearfulness and in the self-distrust which is so often a product of the obsessional experiences.

In some instances the distinction between exposure exercises and behavioural experiments is blurred. The primary purpose of a behavioural experiment is to collect personal, direct information, but the primary purpose of an exposure exercise is to reduce fears and only secondarily to gather fresh information. In order to meet the first purpose of fear-reduction, repeats of the exposure are necessary. Usually the fear declines steadily with planned, systematic exposure exercises.

Direct, personal experience of the decline of the fear during and after exposure exercises is of considerable evidential value. This simple plan structure can be helpful.

Exposure exercises (task described):

1 The purpose of this exposure is to . . . .
2 I predict that I will experience (0–100) fear.
3 Report back: I actually experienced (0–100) fear.
4 I predict that when I repeat this exercise I will experience (0–100).

Supplementary tactics

Obsessional impulses

In addition to these general steps, specific methods may be needed to deal with obsessional impulses, images, and cognitive biases.

Repeated, unwanted, and repugnant impulses, usually of a violent or obscene nature, are prone to cause considerable fear, shame, guilt, and self-distrust. The impulses are often regarded as dangerous and the person feels on the edge of losing control. They regard themselves as unsafe. Avoidance behaviour is the result.

These cognitions need to be explored and then placed against an analysis of whether or not the patient has ever displayed dangerous, objectionable, or unsafe behaviour (rarely, if ever). Care should be taken to explore the possibility that the patient may be subject to thought–action fusion (TAF), in which the occurrence of unwanted ideas, and especially unwanted impulses, are regarded as being almost equivalent, psychologically and/or morally, to the act itself.

For example, a mother who experienced an obsessional impulse to suffocate her 8-month-old infant was extremely distressed by the thought that she might have come close to harming the child. She feared that deep down she may be harbouring violent urges, and that there was an uncontrolled evil streak in her personality. After detailed analysis, it emerged that the patient (typical in these cases) was exceptionally caring and gentle, and had never acted aggressively. Moreover, she was an excellent mother and a devoted, dependable caregiver. She had been consistently kind and was a safe and dependable person. Throughout the exploration and analysis, attention was drawn to the contrast between her consistently safe and kind behaviour and her fleetingly violent intrusive thoughts. Thought and action were prised apart. The patient and therapist compiled written records of the significant contrasts between her consistent behaviour and her unwanted intrusive impulses. These were subsequently used by the patient as prompts and reminders. After the identification of the problem, provision of corrective information, and separation of thought and action, the patient was encouraged to engage in self-directed exercises. She was encouraged to note other examples of TAF and subject them to the same form of cognitive separation. The patient carried out the exercises skilfully and with diligence, and gained strength steadily. She learned to recognize and separate the maladaptive fusions and derived relief and benefit. Her guilt and self-distrust declined and she regarded herself as a safe person and a dependable caregiver.

In assisting the person to make the necessary distinctions between thoughts and actions, the therapist should be careful to avoid entering into rambling metaphysical discussions about the connections, and also bear in mind that in some religions certain kinds of thoughts are indeed regarded as acts of blasphemy. As described earlier, TAFs can be distinguished from religious beliefs, and people with no significant religious beliefs also experience TAFs. Many people who accept the religious view that certain kinds of thoughts are morally equivalent to actions, do not agree that the unwanted thoughts and impulses that are typical of obsessions fall into the same category. They can make the distinction between obsessional ideas and religious beliefs. No special connection between particular religions and the incidence of OCD has been found.

Some obsessions have a superstitious quality to them and it may be necessary to spend some time distinguishing between obsessional ideas and superstitions. For example, very many people feel uncomfortable or would entirely refrain from putting down on paper the thought that harm might come to a friend or relation. While recognizing that in fact, and in logic, writing out the thought on a sheet of paper does not increase the probability of the named person experiencing a misfortune, most people, are nevertheless reluctant to put pen to paper in this way. In the case of obsessional impulses, however, the connection made by the affected person is more intense and less open to rational reconsideration. It seems probable that the distress and reluctance that people with obsessional problems experience is related to their inflated sense of responsibility, and writing down a harmful thought would effectively overload their already exaggerated sense of responsibility; hence the action of writing or thinking a harmful thought is strenuously avoided. As people who experience impulses tend to avoid potentially 'dangerous' places and people, graded and gradual exposure exercises can play a valuable part in treatment.

Obsessional images

Repeated, intrusive, upsetting images can be the major problem (as in the case of a patient who suffered from intrusive images of her friends covered in blood), or an accompaniment of obsessional thoughts/impulses. The images can be extremely distressing, but on average they are less tormenting and briefer than obsessional thoughts. They are relatively easy to dissolve on particular occasions but their repeated return, day after day, is a source of frustration, annoyance, and distress. Recurrent, unacceptable images are prominent in sexual obsessions. Incestuous images are particularly disturbing.

As with all obsessions, exploration of the significance of the image/s is a necessary first step. Attempts are made to defuse any excessive or inappropriate significance which the person attaches to the occurrence or content of the images. The patient's attempts to put right, resist, cancel, or neutralize the image are discouraged. Instead, emphasis is placed on dismissing them as noise in the system.

If there is evidence of inflated responsibility for the images or their moral/psychological consequences, the concept of inflated responsibility should be explained and analysed for the particular patient, paying attention to the universality of the phenomenon of uninvited and unwanted intrusive images.

Post-event processing

The tendency to dwell on upsetting events, to go over them again and again, is particularly prominent in social phobias (Clark and Wells 1995), but also arises in obsessions. Patients are encouraged to refrain from post-event processing because it recalls past distress and failures, thereby sustaining the negative impact of the obsession. It is a self-defeating activity.

The qualities of the different classes of obsessions and how to deal with them

The content of most obsessions falls into three categories, alone or combined: intrusive and unacceptable sexual thoughts, intrusive, unacceptable thoughts of harming others, and intrusive, unacceptable blasphemous thoughts. A unique quality of sexual obsessions is that many of these thoughts are preceded or accompanied by intrusive bodily sensations that are interpreted as signs of sexual arousal or desire. Of course when these sensations are experienced in the wrong place or with the wrong person, and are taken to indicate sexual arousal, the sufferer's reaction can be distressing, shameful, frightening. The problem can be compounded when the patient has become anxious in an inappropriate context (say, near children) and mistakenly interprets the signs of anxiety as those of sexual arousal. It is no wonder that a person caught in this cycle vigorously avoids situations and people where the sensations are evoked. As a further twist, patients can fall into reverse reasoning, for example, 'the fact that I am anxious in the presence of children proves that I am weird and untrustworthy'.

For these reasons, a careful and progressive series of exposure exercises is necessary. The significance of any sensations experienced needs to be clarified, with particular attention to the similarities and differences between the sensations of anxiety and those of sexual arousal. Fears of loss of control are often encountered and these too need to be addressed and disconfirmed in the course of the exposure exercises.

The sexual thoughts often have a visual component. Imagery can be prominent and important. Given the occurrence of unacceptable sexual imagery, an analysis of the significance of sexual imagery is necessary, and it may also be necessary to press the need to forgo attempts at suppressing the unacceptable thoughts and images. Such attempts at suppression can produce paradoxical increases in the images.

Blasphemous obsessions generally take the form of obscene remarks, images, or gestures, often in holy places or during religious services, public or private. Examples include thinking obscene thoughts in church, images of making sexual gestures towards religious figures, images of sex with religious figures, blasphemous thoughts intruding into prayers. These obsessions produce guilt and self-doubt, and can lead to fear of losing one's religion, of being punished, of being sent to eternal hell. Some patients interpret their obsessions as the devil's work, and can even feel that they have become possessed. (In these instances, the therapist needs to remain attentive to the possibility of hallucinations or delusions, however rare in these cases.)

Questions of a religious character can arise (e.g. what is the exact nature and purpose of prayer?) and the patient is encouraged to seek advice from the relevant priest, vicar, rabbi, etc. With the permission of the patient, discussions between the therapist and religious authority are advisable. As the thrust of the therapy is to encourage an adaptive, benign interpretation of the intrusive thoughts, an apparent overlap with religious interpretations can occur. However, it is usually easy for the therapist and religious authority to sort out the differences in a manner that directly benefits the patient.

Patients can become confused, notably in absorbing the concept of morality TAF. In addition to the probability TAF (my thoughts of harm actually increase the risks), the morality TAF refers to the perceived moral equivalence of an unacceptable thought and an unacceptable act. Are unwanted, intrusive obscenities truly blasphemous or are they better regarded as an unsettling psychological phenomenon? The thoughts are by definition unwanted and hence, resisted and rejected. They are ego-dystonic. Blasphemous acts are chosen, purposeful, and in keeping with the person's views and personality.

In treatment, the person's actual behaviour—almost invariably considerate, compassionate, and kind and believing—is contrasted with the intrusions. Attention is drawn to the views of relatives and friends, and the patient may carry out a 'mini-survey' to ascertain whether these friends see them as a kind and convinced believer or a blasphemous oaf. Attention is also drawn to the view expressed by the religious authority, and to the fact that even famous religious figures suffered from blasphemous obsessions. If the religious obsessions have generated avoidance behaviour, such as avoiding church/prayers/events, then a return to the earlier and desired behaviour is encouraged.

The harm obsessions tend to be complex but not therefore the most difficult to tackle. They can be complex because of the potential mixture of a cognitive bias in the form of probability TAF, inflated responsibility, and fear of losing control. The fear of losing control produces maladaptive avoidance behaviour that needs to be reversed. The occurrence of TAF requires a full account of the role of cognitive biases and their unsupportability, coupled with behavioural experiments that enable the patient to test the validity of the TAF. Inflated responsibility has pervasive effects and may underpin the patient's misinterpretations of these thoughts; progress can be facilitated when patients recognize the inflated, exaggerated nature of their perceived responsibility and redraw their 'map' of responsibility to more realistic, acceptable levels.

Thoughts on holidays and holidays from thoughts

Many patients complain of an increase in obsessions during holidays and weekends. When they are not mentally engaged, the intrusive thoughts sneak in and can ruin a holiday. Hence, holiday periods of inactivity and solitude are not recommended; their holidays tend to be packed with activities. Indeed, active and engaging options are preferred. Obsessions tend to occupy empty mental spaces.

In the treatment programme, it is often desirable to encourage the patient to sample the peace that can be gained by taking a 'holiday' from their constant vigilance and their unceasing battles with the obsessions. (Note that a holiday from obsessions is not to be regarded as a blank period, unfilled by any form of planned, deliberate mental activity. A holiday from obsessions should provide an opportunity to substitute desirable, productive activities.) The main cognitive conclusion drawn from declaring a thought holiday is that nothing unfortunate takes place. 'No catastrophe occurred when I refrained from scanning, blocking, and suppressing these thoughts.' The value of these thought holidays is underscored by the resistance that patients initially express when asked to refrain from the scanning and blocking for a prescribed period. They fear that if they do refrain, do go 'off-duty', something horrible may happen (lose control? go crazy?). However, when they do take a thought holiday the effects can be highly beneficial and disconfirm their fearful beliefs. If the patient expresses strong concerns and resistance, the therapist can grade it in slowly, beginning with brief thought holidays in the sessions, then say 10 min out of session, gradually rising to longer periods.

Some patients are well aware that they are vulnerable to obsessions when they are unoccupied. The tactics they adopt can be helpful and even constructive but the use of 'fillers' is not helpful. These fillers are jingles, supposedly reassuring words or phrases, lucky tunes or sayings, and are used in a futile attempt to block out the obsessions. They can, alas, become part of the problem and some patients end up believing that they are no longer able to function unless they use the fillers to block their thoughts. Like all forms of thought blocking it is frustrating and self-defeating and should be discouraged.

CHAPTER 8

How to assess progress and deal with problems

The primary aim of the treatment is to achieve a decrease in the frequency of the obsessions and in the distress that they produce. In theory, it is possible to eliminate the obsessions, and in practice this is achieved in many but not all cases. Given that the cause of the obsessions is the person's catastrophic misinterpretation of the significance of their unwanted, intrusive thoughts, it follows that if this cause is removed then the obsessions should end. If the person reinterprets the intrusive thoughts as benign events, which are neither threatening nor personally damaging, the obsessions should diminish and then disappear.

In practice, changes in interpretation of what had been a dominating feature of the person's daily life, are seldom abrupt and complete. Rather, the person's interpretations change in a gradual and erratic fashion; sometimes the person experiences changes in the degree of conviction or the believability of the interpretations rather than a complete switch to a fresh interpretation. So the therapist, and patient, should aim for a fundamental shift in interpretation and the total elimination of the obsessions, but both may settle for a substantial decline in frequency and distress.

How then is progress assessed? The regular reports made by the patient reveal both frequency and distress and are therefore of paramount importance. The reports are an essential measure of progress and provide the basis for the self-correcting aspect of the treatment. The patient's recordings are supplemented by those of the therapist. Not treatment programme is satisfactory unless and until the frequency and distress scores come way down, to within tolerable, even normal, levels. In the short term, significant reductions in frequency and distress are sufficient signs of improvement, but for the longer term, more is needed. Broader changes are necessary in order to consolidate the improvements.

Evidence of important changes in the interpretation of intrusive thoughts is needed. Have the causes of the obsessions been dealt with? The regular scores reported by the patient on the Personal significance scale are necessary evidence.

At the conclusion of therapy these scores must be supplemented by the patent's responses during the re-administration of all of the pretreatment measures— the Obsessive-Compulsive Inventory (OCI), Yale Obsessive-Compulsive Scale (Y-BOCS, especially the obsessions subscore), the Beck Depression Inventory (BDI), and so on, plus the full structured interview (preferably completed by someone other than the therapist). An important index of change is the patient's behaviour. Evidence of persistent avoidance behaviour, including concealment, neutralization etc., are of course signs of difficulty. The full list of measures used in assessing progress is as follows.

1 Session-by-session changes:
   (a) patient's diary recordings (frequency, distress);
   (b) patient's weekly assessment of obsessional activity;
   (c) therapist's assessment, each session;
   (d) patient's personal significance scores, at the start of each session;
   (e) qualitative reports of reduced avoidance (social, concealment, neutralizing);
   (f) qualitative reports of enhanced social and other behaviour;
   (g) qualitative reports of enhanced mood;
   (h) qualitative reports of enhanced concentration.

2 Post-treatment status:
   (a) all of the session-by-session changes need to be incorporated in this assessment;
   (b) structured interview and Y-BOCS, preferably completed by someone other than the therapist;
   (c) psychometrics (OCI, BDI, PSS);
   (d) behaviour tests;
   (e) TAF scale.

Problems

The most significant problems are those that arise from attempts to change the patient's catastrophic misinterpretations: according to the cognitive theory, these misinterpretations are the cause of the obsession and hence, must be dealt with. In some cases the misinterpretations prove to be inflexible and persist unchanged despite the educational or other components of treatment. A second and related problem is encountered when the patient gradually endorses a more benign interpretation of their intrusive thoughts within the sessions, but in some outside situations remains as convinced as ever that the intrusive thoughts are dangerous or damaging or uniquely revealing. This gulf can be difficult to overcome. In tackling both of these problems—inflexible misinterpretations and non-generalizing changes in interpretations—the use of behavioural experiments can be extremely helpful.

As mentioned earlier, in attacking obsessions, and other forms of psychological disorders, the most powerful and persuasive methods of change are direct, personal experiences. They carry far greater evidential weight for the patient than do reams of statistics and 'cold' technical information about obsessions in general. Information about the number of people who experience unwanted, intrusive thoughts or who suffer from the disorder, etc., is helpful but rarely sufficient.

By setting up behavioural experiments that test important beliefs (e.g. I will make obscene remarks, people will reject me if . . . , etc.), the patient is given opportunities to collect direct, personal evidence relevant to the specific beliefs. A systematic series of such mini-experiments can be powerful and help to overcome interpretation problems in therapy. It is useful to have the patient write down their *specific* expectations of what will happen, and then record the disconfirmations (usual) or confirmations (rare).

Similarly, changes in behaviour (especially reductions in avoidance) can have a major impact on beliefs and interpretations. Quite often it is the combination of these two tactics—behavioural experiments and reducing avoidance behaviour—that leads to changes in misinterpretations. The patient is encouraged to describe and predict (preferably in writing) what will happen if the avoidance behaviour, such as neutralizing, is stopped. A suitable behavioural experiment is devised and the patient engages in the required behaviour, recording the results. After each test, conclusions are drawn.

Some common questions are: 'What will happen if I refrain from suppressing the thoughts?', 'What will happen if I refrain from trying to put right, to correct, the thoughts?', 'What will happen if I resume attending church?', 'What will happen if I tell my parents about my thoughts?'

Some misinterpretations are slower to change than others. Beliefs that people will reject one if they learn about the obsessions tend to shift more slowly because the ideas and attitudes of other people are not directly accessible in the same way as one's self-appraisals. The cognition, 'I am a wicked immoral person' is directly accessible but, 'They will think badly of me, that I am wicked' is not so accessible, nor is the relevant information.

Obsessive-compulsive disorder (OCD) and depression are often associated and many patients with obsessions are or have been depressed. The recurrence or exacerbation of depression can interfere with treatment but should not preclude it. Obviously, any steps taken to reduce the depression are recommended. Similarly, co-morbid social phobia can hamper treatment and if so, needs to be dealt with simultaneously.

Practically speaking, many patients with accompanying depression are taking medication, and changes in drugs or dosage levels are not infrequently associated with emotional turbulence. At times it is necessary to slow therapy until the patient's emotional state or mood is stable. Typically, these episodes of emotional disturbance retard progress but do not have a lasting adverse effect on improvements already made in overcoming the maladaptive misinterpretations of one's intrusive thoughts.

It scarcely needs mentioning, but the patient's life circumstances play a major part in the persistence of the problem. Retreating into solitude and seclusion, avoiding human contact, having no regular work, no close relationships—all of those familiar patterns serve to deepen the misery and also to ensure that the catastrophic misinterpretations are conserved. The usual attempts to restore the patient to a more gratifying and fulfilling everyday life should not be neglected.

Follow-up and prevention

At the end of treatment it is important to remind patients that unwanted intrusive thoughts are a universal experience and that they will only become obsessional if misinterpreted as having catastrophic meaning. Hence, the patient is advised to continue regarding the thoughts as benign and neither dangerous nor uniquely revealing. They are encouraged to collect and evaluate the reasons for their interpretations of any newly troubling thoughts, to block the temptation to avoid, to forgo attempts to suppress the unwanted thoughts, to refrain from neutralizing and concealment. In general, if they use the methods they have acquired during therapy they should be well equipped to deal with any threatened recurrence.

Follow-up evaluations can be scheduled for intervals of 1 month, 3 months, 6 months, and 1 year, with more frequent consultations if necessary.

Therapist's toolkit

Contents

Toolkit form 1: Semi-structured interview on obsessions

1. Give me a full description of each of the troubling thoughts that keep coming into your mind against your wishes (quote patient's exact words whenever possible).

   (a)

   (b)

   (c)

2. When, and how often, do you have each (a), (b), and (c)?

3. What sets them off? (a), (b), and (c)

   Originally, was there a particular moment/event when they began?

4. Do they affect:

   (a) your concentration?

   (b) your mood?

   (c) your work?

5. How do you attempt to deal with them?

   5a. Do you resist them? What will happen if you do not resist them?

6. What helps you to deal with these thoughts?

7. What fails to help you with these thoughts?

8. When did the first of these thoughts begin?

   (a) Why do you think these thoughts began in the first place?

   (b) Did you keep them secret—if so why?

9. Have you told anyone else about these thoughts? (details please)

10. How did they react?

11. Why do the thoughts keep coming back?

12. Do these thoughts tell you anything about yourself—what kind of person you are?

13. Has it changed the way you behave towards other people?

14. Has is changed the way other people behave towards you?

15. What will happen if you stop trying to cancel out the thoughts, block them, or fight against them?

16. Do you keep a close watch on these thoughts? Do you constantly monitor them?

    16a. What would happen if you stopped monitoring the thoughts in this way?

17. Have you ever acted out one of these thoughts? (details please)

18. Have these thoughts ever made you feel crazy, or about to go crazy? (details please)

19. Have you ever felt that you might lose control and do something danger-ous or weird? (details please)

20. Do the thoughts make you feel that you cannot be trusted?

21. If your thoughts are about harming other people, do they focus on par-ticular people?

22. Why do they focus on these particular people?

23. Have you ever had similar harmful thoughts about any strong and confident person?

24. Most obsessions fall into one of three categories—aggressive thoughts, unacceptable sexual thoughts, and anti-religious thoughts—which group do your obsessions fall into?

25. Why don't you have obsessions about the other categories?

26. Do your obsessions make you feel:
    (a) bad, wicked, or evil?
    (b) crazy or weird?
    (c) untrustworthy or dangerous?
    (d) other?

27. Are your thoughts related to your moods? Good moods or bad moods?

28. After an upsetting event, do you spend a lot of time going over and over what happened and why?

29. Have you ever received treatment for these distressing thoughts? If yes, when and where?

30. What were the effects? Why did it help, or fail to help you?

Toolkit form 2: Personal significance scale

Please read the following statements carefully and make a mark anywhere on the line to show the extent to which you agree with each statement.
Specific thoughts, impulses, images:

1. Are these thoughts all nonsense or are they significant for you?

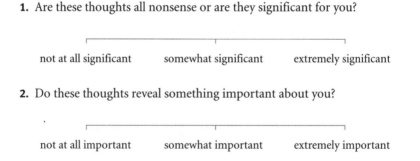

not at all significant   somewhat significant   extremely significant

2. Do these thoughts reveal something important about you?

not at all important   somewhat important   extremely important

3. Are these thoughts a sign that you are original?

```
not at all            somewhat          very original
```

4. Do these thoughts mean that you might lose control and do something awful?

```
not at all             possibly           definitely
```

5. Do these thoughts mean that you are an imaginative person?

```
not at all imaginative   somewhat imaginative   extremely imaginative
```

6. Do these thoughts mean that you might go crazy one day?

```
not at all likely       somewhat likely        very likely
```

7. Is it important for you to keep these thoughts secret from most or all of the people you know?

```
not at all important   somewhat important   extremely important
```

8. Do these thoughts mean that you are a sensitive person?

```
not at all sensitive     somewhat sensitive    extremely sensitive
```

9. Do these thoughts mean that you are a dangerous person?

```
not at all dangerous    somewhat dangerous    definitely dangerous
```

10. Do these thoughts mean that you cannot be trusted?

```
completely trustworthy    somewhat trustworthy    not at all trustworthy
```

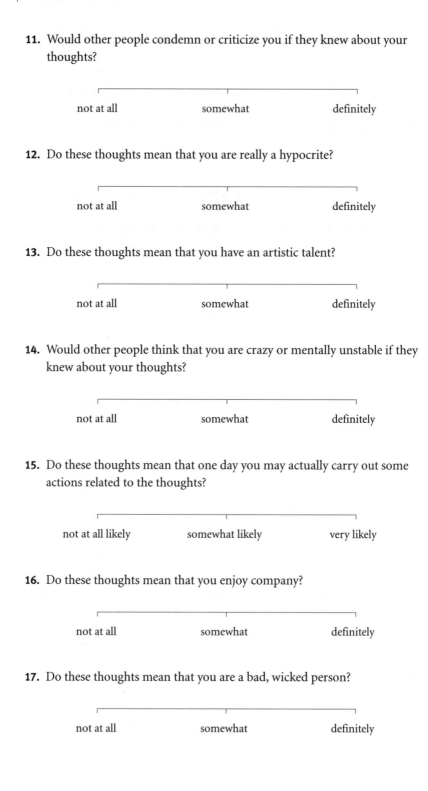

11. Would other people condemn or criticize you if they knew about your thoughts?

not at all	somewhat	definitely

12. Do these thoughts mean that you are really a hypocrite?

not at all	somewhat	definitely

13. Do these thoughts mean that you have an artistic talent?

not at all	somewhat	definitely

14. Would other people think that you are crazy or mentally unstable if they knew about your thoughts?

not at all	somewhat	definitely

15. Do these thoughts mean that one day you may actually carry out some actions related to the thoughts?

not at all likely	somewhat likely	very likely

16. Do these thoughts mean that you enjoy company?

not at all	somewhat	definitely

17. Do these thoughts mean that you are a bad, wicked person?

not at all	somewhat	definitely

18. Do you feel responsible for these thoughts?

        not at all   somewhat   definitely

19. Do you feel that it is important for you to cancel out or block the thoughts?

  not at all important   somewhat important   extremely important

20. Would other people think that you are a bad, wicked person if they knew about your thoughts?

        not at all   somewhat   definitely

21. Do you think that you should avoid certain people or places because of these thoughts?

        not at all   somewhat   definitely

22. Do these thoughts mean that you are weird?

        not at all   somewhat   definitely

23. Do these thoughts mean something else? Please give details:

        not at all   somewhat   definitely

24. Should you fight against and resist these thoughts?

        not at all   somewhat   definitely

25. What caused your thoughts to occur when they started?

26. Why do these thoughts keep coming back?

Toolkit form 3: Unwanted intrusive thoughts
Work sheet

Date: Participant:

The significance of unwanted intrusions

(Therapists: use a fresh sheet for each important unwanted intrusive thought)

1. Statement of most important unwanted intrusive thoughts (UITs), as described by the patient, in the patient's own words.

   (a)

   (b)

2. A statement of the significance that the patient attaches to the UIT, in the patient's own words.

   (a)

   (b)

3. Ask patients to rate how strongly they believe in the interpretations (significance) they attach to the UIT, on a scale from 0 (not at all) to 100 (totally certain that this is correct).

   UIT 1:   (a)   (b)   (c)

   (i)   What are the reasons for this interpretation?

   (ii) What are the reasons against it?

   (iii) What important evidence is missing?

   (iv) How can you collect it? (surveys, behaviour, exposure, etc.)

4. Can you think of some alternative explanations?

5. What would your close friends/relatives think of your interpretations of your thoughts? (details—who, when, etc.)

6. How do they interpret your reported thoughts?

7. If a very close friend of yours reported similar thoughts, what would you think of him/her?

8. How would you interpret his/her thoughts?

9. If a close friend asked you for advice about how to deal with his/her unwanted thoughts, what would you recommend?

10. Why do you conceal your thoughts, if you do?

11. Does this concealment work (help you, harm you)?

   11a. What exactly will happen if you cease to conceal your thoughts?

12. Why do you avoid places/people?

13. Does it work?

   13a. What exactly will happen if you cease to avoid?

14. What methods do you use to prevent the thoughts?

15. Do they work?

   15a. What exactly will happen if you stop preventing the thoughts?

16. What methods do you use to get rid of the thoughts?

17. Do they work?

   17a. What exactly will happen if you stop trying to get rid of the thoughts?

18. How many of your methods of trying to avoid, prevent or remove your UITs have failed?

   18a. Why did each of these fail? (in participant's own words)

   [Therapist: now go on to: (a) Alternative explanations (Toolkit form 11); (b) The reactions of friends Toolkit form 15) (when these two steps are appropriate).]

Toolkit form 4: Measure of obsessional activity

At the beginning of each session collect information about the frequency, etc., of the obsessions in the previous period (usually a week, but can be longer or shorter). NB: the collection of information by means of this questionnaire at the start of every session does not remove the need for the patient to complete the Daily record form.

This questionnaire can be filled out by the patient or used by the therapist to collect and fill in the information.

Obsessional activity (tick one box)

during the past week ☐

during the past month ☐

during the past few days ☐

1. During that past week/month/few days, were your obsessions:

absent	occasional	common	frequent	very frequent
0	25	50	75	100

2. During the past week/month/few days, were your obsessions distressing?

not at all	a little	moderately	very	extremely
0	25	50	75	100

3. During the past week/month/few days, were your obsessions intrusive (i.e. did they disrupt your concentration)?

not at all	a little	moderately	very	extremely
0	25	50	75	100

4. During the past week, how long, on average, did each obsession last?

5. During the past week/month/few days, was the content of your obsessions the same or different from earlier weeks/months?

   Same/Different

   5a. if different content, what has changed?

6. Was this a typical week/month for you? If not, why not?

   6a. Were there any special or unusual events? What? When?

Toolkit form 5: Daily record

(0 = not at all, 50 = moderate, 100 = maximum)

Day	Date	Frequency (0, 1, 2–5, 6–10, 10–50)	Intensity (0–100)	Interfering (0–100)	Upsetting (0–100)

Toolkit form 6: Session-by-session progress chart

Patient:

Session No.

Date:

1. Patient to complete Personal significance scale
2. Collect and discuss patient's Measure of obsessional activity form
3. Complete therapist's version of Measure of obsessional activity form
4. Collect patient's general report-back, including special events, if any
5. Collect the recorded tape, discuss, reload in machine
6. Collect specific report-back on homework tasks:
   (a) exposure exercises;
   (b) behavioural experiments;
   (c) mini-surveys;
   (d) other.
7. Summarize specific treatment tactics used in this session, plus patient's responses.
8. Prepare plans for homework assignments:
   (a) exposure exercises;
   (b) behavioural experiments;
   (c) mini-surveys;
   (d) other.
9. General progress notes
10. Agenda for next session

Toolkit form 7: Thought–action fusion scale

Do you *disagree* or *agree* with the following statements?

	Disagree strongly	Disagree	Neutral	Agree	Agree strongly
Thinking of making an extremely critical remark to a friend is almost as unacceptable to me as actually saying it	0	1	2	3	4
If I think of a relative/friend losing their job, this increases the risk that they will lose their job	0	1	2	3	4
Having a blasphemous thought is almost as sinful to me as a blasphemous action	0	1	2	3	4
Thinking about swearing at someone else is almost as unacceptable to me as actually swearing	0	1	2	3	4
If I think of a relative/friend being in a car accident, this increases the risk that he/she will have a car accident	0	1	2	3	4
When I have a nasty thought about someone else, it is almost as bad as carrying out a nasty action	0	1	2	3	4

Statement	0	1	2	3	4
If I think of a friend/relative being injured in a fall, this increases the risk that he/she will have a fall and be injured	0	1	2	3	4
Having violent thoughts is almost as unacceptable to me as violent acts	0	1	2	3	4
If I think of a relative/friend falling ill this increases the risk that he/she will fall ill	0	1	2	3	4
When I think about making an obscene remark or gesture in church, it is almost as sinful as actually doing it	0	1	2	3	4
If I wish harm on someone, it is almost as bad as doing harm	0	1	2	3	4
If I think of myself being injured in a fall, this increases the risk that I will have a fall and be injured	0	1	2	3	4
If I think about making an obscene gesture to someone else, it is almost as bad as doing it	0	1	2	3	4

Toolkit form 7 (*Continued*)

	Disagree strongly	Disagree	Neutral	Agree	Agree strongly
If I think of myself being in a car accident, this increases the risk that I will have a car accident	0	1	2	3	4
When I think unkindly about a friend, it is almost as disloyal as doing an unkind act	0	1	2	3	4
If I think of myself falling ill, this increases the risk that I will fall ill	0	1	2	3	4
If I have a jealous thought, it is almost the same as making a jealous remark	0	1	2	3	4
Thinking of cheating in a personal relationship is almost as immoral to me as actually cheating	0	1	2	3	4
Having obscene thoughts in a church is unacceptable to me	0	1	2	3	4

(Source: Shafran *et al.* 1996).

Toolkit form 8: List of unwanted intrusive thoughts (a)

Virtually everyone experiences some unwanted, intrusive thoughts. It is a common human experience. This is a list of thoughts, images, and impulses reported by non-clinical participants and by patients with obsessions.

Intrusive, unwanted thoughts, images, and impulses

1.	*Impulse*	to hurt or harm someone (non-clinical)
2.	*Impulse*	to say something nasty and damning to someone (non-clinical)
3.	*Thought*	of harm to, or death of, close friend or family member (non-clinical)
4.	*Thought*	of acts of violence in sex (clinical)
5.	*Impulse*	to crash car, when driving (clinical)
6.	*Thought*	'Why should they do that? They shouldn't do that', in relation to people 'misbehaving' (non-clinical)
7.	*Impulse*	to attack, or strangle cats or kittens (clinical)
8.	*Thought*	'I wish he/she were dead', with reference to persons close and dear, also other (clinical)
9.	*Thought*	to harm partner with physical violence (clinical)
10.	*Impulse*	to attack and violently punish someone, for example, to throw a child out of a bus (non-clinical)
11.	*Impulse*	to engage in certain sexual practices that involve pain to the partner (non-clinical)
12.	*Thought*	'Did I commit this crime?', when reading or hearing reports of crime (clinical)
13.	*Thought*	that one might go berserk all of a sudden (clinical)
14.	*Thought*	wishing and imagining that someone close to her was hurt or harmed (non-clinical)
15.	*Impulse*	to violently attack and kill a dog (non-clinical)

16.	*Thought*	'These boys when they were young'—a mechanically repeated phrase (clinical)
17.	*Impulse*	to attack or harm someone, especially own son, with bat, knife, or heavy object (clinical)
18.	*Thought*	of unnatural sexual acts (non-clinical)
19.	*Thought*	of hurting someone by doing something nasty, not physical violence, 'Would I or would I not do it?' (non-clinical)
20.	*Impulse*	to be rude and say something nasty to people (non-clinical)
21.	*Thought*	thought of obscene words, with large, clear, images of the words in print (clinical)
22.	*Image*	mental picture of stabbing a passer-by (clinical)
23.	*Image*	mental picture of stripping in church (non-clinical)

(Source: Rachman and deSilva 1978)

List of unwanted, uninvited, intrusive thoughts (b)

Virtually all people experience at least some unwanted and unacceptable thoughts, or images, or impulses. Certain ideas are particularly common. These are some examples of common intrusive ideas:

- an urge to shout or disturb a peaceful gathering
- an urge to attack an animal
- an urge to inflict pain on someone
- an urge to make an obscene gesture
- an urge to harm someone
- an impulse to drive off a bridge
- an urge to act violently
- unacceptable blasphemous thoughts or images
- thoughts of harming a child
- unacceptable sexual thoughts or images
- an impulse to drive into oncoming traffic
- having obscene images
- thoughts of harm coming to a family member
- an impulse to run in front of oncoming traffic
- an urge to say something rude/nasty to someone

- thoughts of unacceptable sexual acts
- an impulse to jump out of a high window
- thoughts of harming a close relative
- repeated thoughts/images of the death of a relative or friend
- an urge to drive into a pedestrian
- repeated senseless thoughts or sounds
- repeated thoughts of losing control
- an urge to make a sexually inappropriate gesture or remark
- repeated worries about one's sexual identity, preference
- repeated bloody, violent images
- an urge to attack someone

Toolkit form 9: An explanation of the treatment

Obsessions are repugnant and unwanted intrusive thoughts. The person resists them but they occur over and over again, interfering with concentration, and are extremely upsetting. Usually, the obsessions are so awful and repugnant that the sufferer feels too ashamed or anxious to tell other people. It can become a shameful secret.

It is important to recognize that virtually everyone regularly experiences thoughts, or images, or impulses that are unwanted. For the most part they are simply ignored or dismissed as nonsensical. However, if the person experiencing such unwanted thoughts interprets them as having importance for them personally, then the thoughts can turn into obsessions. If the person begins to believe that the unwanted thoughts are revealing, important, signs of a mental abnormality, signs of losing control, and so on, then difficulty and stress can develop. We will provide you with a list of commonly experienced unwanted thoughts reported by average people, and a list of thoughts reported by patients with obsessions. The content of the thoughts experienced by patients and average people is similar but the obsessions are more intense, more frequent, and more upsetting.

The purpose of the treatment is to assist you in modifying and normalizing your interpretation of your unwanted and intrusive thoughts. When you achieve this, the obsessions will weaken, cease to upset you, and may even go completely.

Unwanted intrusive thoughts reach a clinically significant level if and when you interpret them as being of great personal meaning. We all have unwanted thoughts but can dismiss them. For example, most drivers will get angry on occasions, and even curse under their breath or openly. However, they seldom take seriously the aggressive feelings they experience while at the wheel. They soon calm down and dismiss their aggressive reactions as unimportant. By contrast, if a driver has a fleeting idea of deliberately running down a pedestrian, for no reason, that can cause problems. If the driver interprets the idea as showing that they harbour homicidal wishes, it becomes very upsetting. Do you ever have silly thoughts while driving? Or at other times? Do you ever have silly, unwanted thoughts about religion, or sex, or aggression? If so, which of these silly thoughts bother you and which do not? Do you know why some thoughts bother you and others do not?

There are three common themes in obsessions: aggression (harm), blasphemy, unnatural/unacceptable sexual themes or urges (e.g. molesting, or doubts about sexual identity). After establishing the category into which your obsessions fall, ask yourself why the other themes do not feature in your obsessions. The contents of your obsessions are closely connected to your values—do you perhaps 'catastrophize' about thoughts/images that bear on your strongest values—and not about 'insignificant' images/thoughts?

The personal meaning you attach to the unwanted thoughts can increase the frequency and distressing quality of the experience. Likewise, when the personal meaning that you attach to an unwanted, intrusive thought is lowered, there will be a decrease in the distress and frequency of the obsessions. Unwanted, intrusive thoughts arise in the first place as a result of stress or anxiety; stress can give rise to a significant increase in the frequency of such unwanted thoughts.

Unwanted thoughts cause distress and it is quite natural to resist them, to fight them off. However, trying to suppress these intrusive thoughts can unfortunately cause them to increase! The harder you try, the worse they become.

Trying to counteract the thoughts, trying to neutralize them can have an adverse effect on the obsessional experience. Neutralizing refers to any attempt made to 'put right', correct, change, or cancel out the obsession. Common examples include: a compulsive act that counters the thought, generally in order to protect someone from harm; deny the thought, fight it away, say a protective prayer or phrase, visually reanimate the victim(s), etc. Much neutralizing takes place internally (mentally) and can require intense concentration, leading to exhaustion. The main forms of external neutralization are compulsive checking, cleaning, and ordering. In the short term, these attempts at neutralization are often successful in reducing a certain amount of anxiety/discomfort, and the effects are typically achieved quite promptly. In the longer term, however, acts of neutralization serve to protect the idea that the thoughts are indeed of great personal meaning and that the distress or the feared event might well have occurred if the patient had failed to carry out the neutralizing act. In fact, the distress that arises from an unwanted intrusive thought will diminish spontaneously, albeit a little more slowly than occurs after a deliberate act of neutralization.

Hence, part of the treatment is designed to help you overcome the strong urge to 'put right', cancel out, or neutralize the thoughts. The major aim is to help you achieve a more realistic, calmer interpretation of the personal meaning of your unwanted thoughts.

Additional reading is available, if requested, including copies of this treatment manual. See also de Silva and Rachman (1998), and for vivid examples of obsessions, Osborn (1998). See also Schwartz (1996) and Foa and Wilson (1991).

Toolkit form 10: Cognitive tactics

1. This thought (or image or impulse) means that:

2. My reasons for believing that meaning are as follows:

3. The specific evidence for believing that meaning is:

4. The reasons for disbelieving that it really means that include the following:

5. The specific evidence for disbelieving that it really means that includes:

6. What do other people who know about your thoughts, for example, friends or relatives, think they mean?

7. Do you know their reasons for thinking so?

8. If you do not have the information from them, are you willing to ask specific people?

These general enquiries are supplemented by specific questions, along the following lines:

- How many times have you had these intrusive, unacceptable/aggressive/sexual/blasphemous thoughts?
- How many times have these intrusive thoughts been followed by acts of aggression (to children, the elderly, etc.), or embarrassment (e.g. shouting obscenities)?
- Or been followed by unacceptable sexual acts?
- Or been followed by sacrilegious acts?

- How many times have you experienced these disturbing sexual/anxious sensations?
- How many times have these sensations been followed by unacceptable acts of aggression/sex?
- How many times have your disturbing images been followed by carrying out the act?
- Have you ever had disturbing dreams about yourself behaving unacceptably or disturbingly badly?
- If so, were the dreams followed by the unacceptable acts you dreamed about?
- Has any doctor said that you are in danger of ending up crazy?

Toolkit form 11: Alternative significance

Possible alternative interpretations of the significance of the intrusive thoughts

1. List some of the possible alternative explanations of the significance of the thoughts, in the patient's own words, if possible:

   Alternative 1

   Alternative 2

   Alternative 3

2. Reasons for:

   Alternative 1

   Alternative 2

   Alternative 3

3. Reasons against:

   Alternative 1

   Alternative 2

   Alternative 3

4. Evidence missing?

   Alternative 1

   Alternative 2

   Alternative 3

5. Can the evidence be collected. If so, how?

   Alternative 1

   Alternative 2

   Alternative 3

Toolkit form 12: The fate of past obsessions

1. When you first experienced your obsessions what did you think they meant?

2. What did you conclude?

3. What did you do about it, if anything?

4. Did it work, did it help you?

5. Did you tell anyone else about it?
   (a) If not, why not?
   (b) If yes, whom?
   (c) What did they say, or do?

6. Have any of your obsessions become less frequent/intense, or even completely gone?
   (a) Which ones?
   (b) When?

(c) Explain why each one decreased.

(d) What do you conclude from their disappearance?

(e) Why did they weaken/go and other obsessions persist?

7. Were any of your past obsessions followed by unacceptable, catastrophic behaviour?

(a) Violent acts?

(b) Unacceptable sexual acts?

(c) Obscene acts

(d) Shouting in public?

(e) Making a nasty scene in church, others?

8. What exactly prevented you from carrying out any of these acts? (The patient's replies can provide incisive questions to be tackled in behavioural experiments.)

Toolkit form 13: Obsessions and past treatments

1. Have you received psychological treatment?

(a) If so, what and when?

(b) Did it help or not?

(c) Explain its effects on you

2. Have you received psychiatric treatment?

(a) If so, what and when?

(b) Did it help or not?

(c) Explain its effects on you

3. Have you received any self-chosen/other treatment, including reading, self-help manuals, etc.?

(a) If so, what and when?

(b) Did it help or not?

(c) Explain its effects on you

Toolkit form 14: Obsessions and moods

1. Are your obsessions related to your moods?

   (a) How?

2. If they are less intense and/or less frequent when you are up and in a happy mood, how can we explain that? (e.g. Does it mean that you are a less mean, immoral, less dangerous person when you are happy?)

3. If they are more intense and/or frequent when you are down, feeling miserable, how can we explain that? (Again, does it mean that you are a less trustworthy person when you are low? That you are less controlled when low, a more immoral person when low?)

Optional behavioural experiment

1. Try for one whole day to convince yourself that your obsessions are very important and very self-revealing.

2. On the next day, try to convince yourself that the obsessions are insignificant, nonsense, mere noise—for an entire day.

3. Compare the intensity and frequency of the obsessions on both days.

4. Compare your mood on both days.

Ask the patient to discuss this question: If there is a connection between the obsessions and changes in mood, what conclusions can you make about the significance/meaning of the obsessions?

Toolkit form 15: Concealment of obsessions

1. Did you conceal your obsessions from other people?

   (a) When and for how long?

   (b) Why?

   (c) Did it help?

2. Whom did you tell?

   (a) When?

   (b) Why?

   (c) How did they react?

(d) Did they attach great significance to your obsessions?

(e) If not, why didn't they do so?

3. Do you expect other people to share your interpretations of the meaning of your obsessions? To attach great significance to them?

(a) Did they?

(b) Did they change their attitude to you?

(c) Did they change their behaviour to you?

4. If no to these last three questions, why not?

Analysing the reactions of friends

1. Have you ever told anyone about this? If yes, whom and when?

(a) Was this person/these people someone whose judgement you respect and trust?

2. Have you concealed these thoughts from most people or a selected few people?

(a) From whom?

(b) Why?

3. How did your friend/relation respond when you told him/her?

(a) Did their behaviour towards you change?

(b) Did they show signs of fearing you?

4. Did they avoid you because of what you told them?

5. Are they reluctant to be alone with you?

6. Do they prevent you from being alone with young children?

7. If their behaviour towards you has not changed, what can you say about the importance that they attach to those thoughts of yours?

Toolkit form 16: Responsibility appraisal

1. Do you feel a special responsibility for making sure that friends and/or relative are safe and protected?

2. Do you make very sure to check that they are safe and well?

3. Do you frequently feel that if some misfortune occurs to one of your friends/relatives you will be responsible?

4. Do you feel specially responsible for checking the safety of your home and everyone and everything in it, before you leave?

5. Do you feel specially responsible for checking the safety of your home and everyone and everything in it, before you go to bed at night?

6. On some occasions, do you feel specially responsible for ensuring that everyone has a good time?

7. Do you feel guilty if you have not made absolutely sure that your family/friends are safe?

8. Do you spend a great deal of time and effort thinking about the safety and well-being of your family and friends?

Toolkit form 17: Behavioural experiment

1. The purpose of the experiment is to test the belief that ....

2. On _____ I will (go to, ask, tell, etc.) the following people/place.

3. I predict that I will (a) feel and (b) do the following:

4. I predict that (another person/people) will do the following:

Report on actual event

1. On _____, I carried out the experiment in/at:

2. I felt _____ , and behaved _____ .

3. The other person/people said_____ and did _____.

4. My predictions were correct/incorrect.

5. My belief that _____ was supported/disconfirmed.

Toolkit form 18: Mini-survey

Patients tend to assume that everyone shares their view of the dangerousness and revealing qualities of intrusive thoughts. They are convinced that everyone will be shocked and reject them.

But, do other people really attach great significance to one's obsessions? Is it true? Collect the evidence. The aim of the mini-survey is to collect evidence about people's thoughts and attitudes, from the people themselves, instead of inferring or merely guessing what other people think or are likely to think.

Ask the patient to select a few people whom they trust and whose opinion they value. It should be agreed in advance that at least a few people will be asked to provide their views; asking only one person can lead to a distorted conclusion. In most instances the mini-survey begins with a question or two about the respondent's own thoughts. 'Do you ever have unwanted, intrusive thoughts or images?' If yes, 'Do you think they are important; do they mean something important about you?' If so, 'What? Why?' And, 'What do you do about them?' 'Have you told anyone else about these thoughts?' 'What did they say or do?'

Now, 'If I told you about some of my unwanted, intrusive thoughts would you be willing to listen?' If yes, go ahead, describe the thoughts and explain that you are trying to overcome them with the help of a psychologist.

Remember the reaction of each person and note whether their behaviour/attitude towards you changes after you have spoken to them. After completing a few such interviews, review the evidence and draw conclusions.

1. Were your expectations of how other people react to your description of your obsessions correct or incorrect?

2. How many people told you about their own unwanted intrusive thoughts?

3. Did you reject them?

4. Were most people willing to listen to your descriptions?

5. Were they understanding?

6. Did they reject or avoid or isolate you?

7. Did their behaviour towards you change?

8. What can you conclude about how other people interpret the meaning of your obsessions?

CHAPTER 10

Case illustrations

Case 1

The first case is that of a 40-year-old man with an 11-year-old daughter and a 7-year-old son. He reported that he was experiencing unwanted intrusive and very distressing thoughts of harm coming to his children, and was performing numerous repetitive acts to protect them. The intrusive thoughts involved someone else harming the children (e.g. being robbed or attacked, or seeing them injured in a disaster or motor accident). His thoughts were vivid and detailed and often took the form of a video-like image. They arose five to six times per day, lasted for up to an hour and were distressing, tiring, and time-consuming. When his wife was pregnant with the first child he experienced a great deal of anxiety about whether the baby would be born healthy. After the birth he became hyper-vigilant for the baby's safety and began to experience intrusive thoughts about family members or strangers hurting the child. Media reports could trigger the thoughts and were vivid, sometimes progressing to scenes of a funeral and a coffin. He developed a technique to block these thoughts and also carried a steak knife when he took the baby for a walk in a stroller.

His method for dealing with the thoughts was to carry out compulsive rituals every time one occurred, for example, squeezing his fists and shouting 'stop' to himself, but this was of minimal effectiveness. His most effective compulsion was to grasp his wristwatch and say; 'they are safe.' The patient felt that if he discontinued his attempts to block the thoughts he would experience severe anxiety.

He refrained from telling anyone about his thoughts because he felt other people might interpret the thoughts as indicating that he was a risk to the safety of his children. He also thought that others would regard him as weird or crazy. Even though he felt that realistically he was a loving and concerned parent, the occurrence of these thoughts made him feel weak and raised the possibility that perhaps he had something on his conscience.

The patient received eight weekly sessions of therapy at the end of which his obsessions had been reduced to no more than one every other week. They were no longer distressing.

His ratings on the Personal significance scale were high before treatment but reduced to close to 0 at the end of treatment. Before treatment he rated the thoughts as extremely important and negative, that they were extremely revealing about him, that it was extremely important to conceal the thoughts from other people, that although he did not regard himself as dangerous he felt that it was somewhat likely that he might go crazy as a result of them. He also endorsed the statement that other people would think of him as mentally unstable if they knew what his thoughts were, and he felt that his thoughts indicated that he was weird. The patient also felt that it was essential to cancel out or block the thoughts. By the end of treatment his scores on the Personal significance scale indicated that he felt the thoughts were not important, not revealing and were not at all likely to make him go crazy one day. He felt that he was not at all dangerous or unstable and that it was no longer necessary to cancel out or block these thoughts. His avoidance behaviour had been eliminated.

On the other pre-assessment scales, his elevated scores on depression and on the Thought–action fusion scale, and obsessional questionnaires, had all been reduced to insignificant levels. Overall, he was significantly less anxious and demoralized and felt liberated by the fact that he no longer had 'a bad little secret' hidden away.

During the course of treatment some difficulties were inevitably experienced. It took him quite a while to accept that everyone experiences unwanted intrusive thoughts because he was convinced that his own thoughts were abnormal and weird. It also took him some time to gather the strength and courage to disclose to family and friends what the thoughts were. He had begun simply by telling them that he had a condition called obsessive-compulsive disorder (OCD) and suffered from intrusive thoughts but he concealed the content. As he became more comfortable he revealed to them that the thoughts concerned harm coming to his children. When he finally was able to disclose to relations and friends, the response that he received was supportive and empathic. He also said that he had received from other people evidence of the fact that he is a dedicated parent and confirmation of the fact that other people also have unwanted intrusive thoughts. At follow-up he remained well.

Case 2

The second illustrative case was more complicated. It was ultimately successful but required 18 sessions. The second patient was a 45-year-old woman who reported a history of obsessional thoughts going all the way back to her teenage years. She reported having roughly 50–60 unwanted intrusive thoughts each day and said that they generally took two forms: those that occurred out of the blue, full blown, and others that unfolded gradually. The intrusive thoughts and images involved acts of violence or disaster, killing, imprisonment, fatal diseases. In roughly 75 per cent of the instances she was the aggressor and in roughly 25 per cent of the images the victim. The thoughts could be triggered by a variety of cues such as media images of violence, perceived mistreatment, driving disputes, and so forth. The thoughts generally ended in imagined catastrophic consequences, such as ending up in prison, losing her husband, or dying. The thoughts were more frequent when she felt stressed or was in a low mood. She tried to resist the thoughts but was not particularly effective in doing so.

She had not disclosed the thoughts to anyone until a few years ago because of her concern that other people would regard her as being mentally abnormal and then treat her differently. In addition she worried about the catastrophic consequences if people knew about her thoughts and that they might begin to avoid her. She felt that the thoughts indicated that she had a capacity for evil, might go crazy one day, and that she was in some way fatally flawed. She was also concerned that she might lose control one day and carry out a repugnant violent act. Because of a high level of background anxiety, progress was erratic. Gradually, however, she began to assemble and evaluate alternative explanations for the thoughts and accumulate evidence that pertained to the various alternative explanations.

She was reluctant to refrain from neutralizing activities because she felt that if she did so it would let her guard down and she might carry out one of the violent acts. Initial attempts to assist in curtailing the neutralization were of little effect until she agreed to use the tactic of a 'thought holiday'. During the holiday period, which began with only a limited period of one hour per episode, she gradually began to recognize that so far from increasing her anxiety and feelings of losing control, during the holiday periods in which she refrained from monitoring her thoughts or trying to block them, her anxiety diminished and she felt more in control and calmer. As a natural follow-on, attention was directed towards her constant vigilance and monitoring of her thoughts. Progressively she was able to give up the internal scanning of her thoughts and as a result was less tense and less tired. The difficulties encountered in treatment included persistent avoidance of a variety of social situations in which she felt she might behave inappropriately because of the thoughts, and a festering realistic problem with a troublesome neighbour. The avoidance behaviour was dealt with by planned and gradual exposure exercises, and the dispute with the neighbour was partly resolved. When these difficulties had been dealt with she continued to make good progress and by the end of the 18th session felt that there was no need for further treatment. She said that she had experienced a fundamental shift in the way she viewed her thoughts and the world. In particular she was no longer filtering and interpreting all the information coming from the external world for its threatening and violent qualities. Her doubts about her trustworthiness and general character had also diminished. On the Personal significance scale large decreases were reported in the importance attached to the intrusive thoughts, the probability that she would lose control or carry out a horrific act, the belief that people would reject her if they knew what her thoughts were, and that they would think of her as mentally unstable, and so forth. The substantial decreases in the excessive significance that she had been attaching to the thoughts occurred in parallel with the signs of general clinical progress.

Case 3

This illustrates the treatment of a patient who was tormented by incessant sexual obsessions. A 30-year-old woman sought treatment for her fear that she might anger or offend people by touching them in a sexual, inappropriate manner. She was convinced that this made her a weird, untrustworthy, and bad person.

She attributed the origin of her obsessions to several anxiety-provoking sexual experiences that occurred when she was a young child. She reported memories of several interactions with other young children that seemed inappropriate now that she is an adult. At least one of these events, involving seemingly normative sexual exploration, resulted in reprimands from her mother and left her feeling ashamed.

In order to relieve the anxiety triggered by the obsessions, she compulsively reviewed her actions in order to assure herself she had not committed offensive acts. She reported that her compulsive replaying of events often lasted for hours at a time, especially when returning home alone after being out in public. The patient repeatedly asked her husband for reassurance. When she became extremely distressed she occasionally requested reassurance from the target person, or even from strangers. The patient avoided going out to populated places, and stood as far back as possible from other people.

The obsessions occurred daily and interfered with her ability to work and socialize. The patient was mildly depressed and described some thought–action fusion that was limited to sexual and violent thoughts. The patient recognized that attempts to suppress or neutralize her obsessions increased her anxiety and predicted that attempts to stop suppressing or neutralizing the obsessions would also decrease her distress.

She was given 12 sessions of cognitive behaviour therapy (CBT) directed at deflating the maladaptive interpretations that she was placing on her intrusive thoughts. As gauged from her pretreatment and post-treatment scores on the Personal significance scale, all of her over-interpretations were reduced. The occurrence of obsessions was reduced to a frequency of roughly two or three thoughts per fortnight, and they no longer produced distress. Her depression scores subsided to normal levels, she was active and more sociable again, carrying out voluntary work as a prelude to returning to her job.

Case 4

A 30-year-old self-employed bookkeeper referred himself for treatment of an obsessional disorder, having failed to benefit from a variety of previous treatments, both psychiatric and psychological. He complained of three main obsessions: thoughts and images of harming himself, thoughts of hurting other people, and unwanted sexual thoughts and images. The obsession of causing harm to children was the most distressing and generally focused on his 5-year-old nephew. He described a recent example when he took his nephew out for a drive and had thoughts of 'beating him up and dumping him in the side of the road'. He also had thoughts of harming children who were unfamiliar to him, saying that these can be triggered by driving past a school or seeing children in a playground. He also had occasional thoughts of harming members of his family. His images of self-harm took two main forms. The first involved slashing his wrists, arms, and hands with a knife. The image usually lasted for 15–30s and was triggered by the sight of sharp objects. The second image/thought involved placing his hand on a hot element when cooking on the stove. He also reported unwanted sexual thoughts but said that the associated images were not as intense as those involving aggressive themes.

He reported having the harm images about three times a week and the thoughts of self-harm four to five times a day. The thoughts and images disturbed his concentration and ability to perform his work. He was depressed, and slower than he used to be when performing tasks, partly because he had to repeat things so many times when he lost track of what he was doing. He tried to deal with the obsessions by deliberately thinking of more pleasant things but had little success with this method. He vigorously resisted the images of harming his children, but despite this, they persisted.

The patient attributed the beginning of the obsessions to a stressful period in his life 5 years earlier. He had been working excessively and was feeling very unhappy and embittered. As a result he was drinking a great deal and smoking 'a fair bit of pot'. He said that although he has no strong religious convictions, he does believe in spiritual forces and worried that he might have become possessed.

He concealed his thoughts from everyone else because he expected that others would find them unacceptable and conclude that there was something wrong with him. Despite these fears he felt that he is 'basically a good person'. However, he was extremely worried that he might be going crazy and losing his mental stability. He was particularly worried that the intense anxiety might one day cause him to 'lose control and snap'.

The patient did not perceive himself as being dangerous or weird, but definitely felt that he was different from others and might be 'losing his mind'. He was troubled by the origin of the thoughts and repeatedly questioned himself and the therapist about 'where the thoughts come from', even while acknowledging that everyone has unwanted thoughts. Because they were so foreign to him, the doubts about whether he was 'possessed by some evil spirit' persisted.

He completed the 12-session course of treatment and reported reductions in the personal significance of the thoughts, but they remained at an unacceptably high level. The three key cognitions were that the thoughts are extremely important, that they are personally revealing about him, and that they were a sign that he might go crazy. All of these thoughts originally were endorsed as between 60 and 80 per cent certain and at the termination of treatment they had declined to between 30 and 45 per cent. There was a corresponding decrease in the frequency and intensity of the obsessions but they persisted, albeit at lower levels of intensity and frequency.

In summary, he experienced a moderate improvement in his obsessional disorder, but not sufficient for him to be free of its shackles. It was not clear why he had not made a full improvement, having completed all of the components of the treatment in a cooperative manner. He appeared to benefit most from behavioural retraining, which involved graded and increasingly prolonged contacts with children in public places, but his fears of insanity proved to be resistant. Evidence for and against this interpretation was collected, assessed, and discussed during several sessions but without the ultimate shift that both the therapist and patient had been hoping for. According to him, being mentally disturbed was shown by the fact that he was so unfocussed, indecisive, emotional, and irrational. In support of this interpretation he said he was drifting, didn't know what to do with his life, had no plans, couldn't make decisions, and worked erratically. Evidence against the interpretation was that he was able to take care of himself and communicate with others, keep in touch with his family, and so forth. Although it was not explicitly included in the evidence in favour of the interpretation, the patient was troubled by the fact that his brother had had prolonged admissions to a long-stay psychiatric hospital for mental illness, probably schizophrenia. The patient did not feel that he had any of the symptoms that his brother had displayed, or explicitly state that he was fearful of developing schizophrenia, but he was extremely uneasy about his brother's condition.

Case 5

A 22-year-old woman sought treatment for obsessions that had started to occur 8 months earlier after reading a verse in the bible concerning the sin of blasphemy. She recalled a specific incident at about this time in which she was told that if the Holy Spirit is not in your heart then you would go to hell. She reported a total conviction, with 100 per cent confidence, that the Holy Spirit had indeed left her heart as a result of actions she engaged in during her teenage years. She was unable to describe the specific acts, or to recall them with any kind of certainty, but felt sure that God had not forgotten. Her evidence for the conviction that the Holy Spirit had permanently left her is that she no longer experienced the feeling of joy and peace in her heart. She also said that during prayers she felt she was not in contact with God. In addition she worried that the obsessions might lead her to do unholy or sinful acts. These and related ideas often were accompanied by troubling images of the Devil and the possibility of engaging in wicked behaviour. Indeed she said that her obsessions made her feel bad, wicked, evil, crazy, weird, and occasionally dangerous to herself and to others. She felt that she would continue to be troubled by the obsessions unless and until she experienced a return of the Holy Spirit. The obsessions interfered with her concentration, made her depressed, and had prevented her from attending church and praying in the way in which she had formerly engaged. She had previously had psychological and psychiatric treatment but with little benefit.

The treatment rationale was explained to her and she agreed to participate in the treatment providing that she was given a reassurance that it would not interfere with her faith and religious practices. She attended the first two sessions and reasonable progress appeared to have been made, but she failed to keep her third appointment on the grounds that she had become severely depressed. It was also then learned that 2 years earlier she had been admitted to hospital during a psychotic episode that had responded moderately well to medication. When asked about previous treatments during the initial assessment she had failed to mention this earlier problem or the fact that she was still under medication for that episode and was also receiving medication for a significant bout of depression. In any event, a significant increase in her depression made further participation in the treatment impossible.

It should not be concluded from this unfortunate case that a previous history of serious illness necessarily precludes the use of a cognitive behavioural treatment designed to deal with obsessions; however, the prognosis in such cases cannot be optimistic.

Case 6

A 25-year-old salesman complained of persistent intrusive thoughts of harming other people, especially pedestrians. He was continually checking to determine whether or not he had caused harm to other people and was drowning in self-doubt. He also complained that he felt exceptionally responsible for caring for his friends, family, and relative strangers. He rated the intrusive thoughts about harming others as being extremely important, possibly revealing that he had some deep-lying and concealed aggression, that he was weak and untrustworthy.

The main thrust of treatment was the collection and evaluation of evidence for and against the significance that he was attaching to the intrusive thoughts. This core part of the treatment progressed as planned and resulted in steadily decreasing ratings in the personal significance of the intrusive thoughts, until at the end of the 12-session course of treatment, his ratings of their personal significance had reduced from roughly 80 per cent to as low as 5 per cent. The treatment was supplemented by response prevention of his overt checking behaviour, which he carried out to ensure that he had not harmed anyone. On this part of the treatment he also progressed steadily and successfully. The final component of the treatment was to help him to bring about a deliberate reduction in the range and intensity of his perceived responsibility for caring for and protecting other people. By the conclusion of treatment it had reached realistic levels.

In sum, he progressed well through the course of treatment and reported a steady decline in his original own interpretation of the significance of his thoughts. Correspondingly, by the end of treatment he was virtually free of obsessions. At the 6 month follow-up period, there was no recurrence of the obsessions.

References

Abramowitz, J. (1997). Effectiveness of psychological and pharmacological treatments for OCD: a quantitative review. *Journal of Consulting and Clinical Psychology* **65**, 44–52.

Amir, N., Freshman, M., Ramsey, B., Neary, E. and Brigidi, B. (2001). Thought–action fusion in individuals with OCD symptoms. *Behaviour Research and Therapy* **7**, 765–76.

Arkes, H.R. (1981). Impediments to accurate clinical judgment and possible ways to minimize their impact. *Journal of Consulting and Clinical Psychology* **49**, 323–30.

Arntz, A., Rauner, M. and van den Hout, M. (1995). 'If I feel anxious, there must be danger': ex-consequential reasoning in inferring danger in anxiety disorders. *Behaviour Research and Therapy* **33**, 917–25.

Beck, A.T. (1976). *Cognitive therapy and the emotional disorders.* New York: International University Press.

Beck, A.T. (1998). Personal communication. World Congress of Behavioural and Cognitive Psychotherapies, Copenhagen.

Brown, T., Di Nardo, P. and Barlow, D. (1994). *Anxiety Disorders Interview Schedule,* San Antonio, Texas: Psychological Corporation.

Butler, G. and Mathews, A. (1987). Anticipatory anxiety and risk perception. *Cognitive Therapy and Research* **11**, 551–65.

Clark, D.A. and Ball, S. (1991). An experimental investigation of thought suppression. *Behaviour Research and Therapy* **29**, 253–7.

Clark, D.A. and Purdon, C. (1995). The assessment of unwanted intrusive thoughts: a review and critique of the literature. *Behaviour Research and Therapy* **33**, 967–76.

Clark, D.M. (1986). A cognitive approach to panic. *Behaviour Research and Therapy* **24**, 461–70.

Clark, D.M. (1988). A cognitive model of panic. In S. Rachman and J. Maser (eds), *Panic: psychological perspectives.* Erlbaum, Hillsdale, New Jersey, pp. 71–90.

Clark, D.M. (1996). Panic disorder: from theory to therapy. In P.M. Salkovskis (ed.), *Frontiers of cognitive therapy.* New York: Guilford Press, pp. 318–44.

Clark, D.M. (1997). Panic disorder and social phobia. In D.M. Clark and C. Fairburn (eds), *The science and practice of cognitive behaviour therapy.* Oxford: Oxford University Press, pp. 119–54.

Clark, D.M. and Fairburn, C. (Eds) (1997). *The science and practice of cognitive behaviour therapy.* Oxford: Oxford University Press.

Clark, D.M. and Wells, A. (1995). A cognitive model of social phobia. In R. Heimberg, M.R. Liebowitz, D.A. Hope, and F.R. Schneier (eds), *Social phobia: diagnosis, assessment and treatment.* New York: Guilford Press.

Craske, M. (1999). *Anxiety disorders.* Boulder, Colorado: Westview Press, pp. 69–93.

Dadds, M., Gaffney, L.R., Kenardy, J., Oei, T.P. and Evans, L. (1993). An exploration of the relationship between expression of hostility and the anxiety disorders. *Journal of Psychiatric Research* **27**, 17–26.

Dawes, R.M., Faust, D. and Meehl, P.E. (1989). Clinical versus actuarial judgment. *Science* **243**, 1668–74.

de Silva, P. (1994). Obsessions and compulsions. In S. Lindsay and G. Powell (eds), *Handbook of adult clinical psychology.* London: Gower Press, pp. 47–87.

de Silva, P. and Rachman, S. (1997). *Obsessive-compulsive disorder: the facts* (2nd edn). Oxford: Oxford University Press.

Ehlers, A. (1993). Somatic symptoms and panic attacks: a retrospective study of learning experiences. *Behaviour Research and Therapy* **31**, 269–78.

Emmelkamp, P. and Aardema, A. (1999). Metacognition, specific OCD beliefs and OC behaviour. *Clinical Psychology and Psychotherapy* **6**, 139–45.

Eysenck, H.J. and Rachman, S. (1965). *The causes and cures of neurosis.* London: Routledge and Kegan Paul.

Foa, E. and Wilson, R. (1991). *Stop obsessing!* New York: Bantam Dell.

Foa, E., Franklin, M. and Kozak, M. (1998a). Psychosocial treatments for OCD: literature review. In R. Swinson, M.A. Antony, S. Rachman, and M.A. Richter (eds), *Obsessive-compulsive disorder: theory, research and treatment.* New York: Guilford Press, pp. 258–76.

Foa, E., Kozak, M., Salkovskis, P., Coles, M. and Amir, N. (1998b). The validation of a new OCD scale: the Obsessive-Compulsive Inventory. *Psychological Assessment* **10**, 206–14.

Freeston, M. and Ladouceur, R. (1997). What do patients do with their obsessive thoughts? *Behaviour Research and Therapy* **35**, 337–48.

Freeston, M.H., Ladouceur, R., Gagnon, F. and Thibodeau, N. (1993). Beliefs about obsessional thoughts. *Journal of Psychopathology and Behavioural Assessment* **15**, 1–21.

Freeston, M.H., Rheaume, J. and Ladouceur, R. (1996). Correcting faulty appraisals of obsessional thoughts. *Behaviour Research and Therapy* **34**, 433–46.

Freeston, M.H., Ladouceur, R., Gagnon, F., Thibodiau, N., Rheaume, J., Letarte, H. *et al.* (1997). Cognitive-behavioural treatment of obsessive thoughts: a controlled study. *Journal of Consulting and Clinical Psychology* **65**, 405–13.

Frost, R. and Steketee, G. (Eds) (2002). *Cognitive approaches to obsessions and compulsions: theory, assessment and treatment.* Oxford: Elsevier.

Gold, D.B. and Wegner, D.M. (1995). Origins of ruminative thought: trauma, incompleteness, nondisclosure, and suppression. Special issue: Rumination and intrusive thoughts. *Journal of Applied Social Psychology* **25**, 1245–61.

Goodman, W., Price, L., Rasmussen, S., Mazuke, C., Fleischman, R., Hill, C. *et al.* (1989). The Yale Brown Obsessive Compulsive Scale. *Archives of General Psychiatry* **46**, 1006–11.

Hodgson, R. and Rachman, S. (1977). Obsessional compulsive complaints. *Behaviour Research and Therapy* **15**, 389–95.

Horowitz, M. (1975). Intrusive and repetitive thoughts after experimental stress. *Archives of General Psychiatry* **32**, 1457–63.

Jaspers, K. (1963). *General psychopathology.* Chicago: Chicago University Press.

Lewis, A. (1936). Problems of obsessional illness. *Proceedings of the Royal Society of Medicine* **29**, 325–36.

Lewis, A. (1966). Obsessional disorder. In R. Scott (ed.), *Price's textbook of the practice of medicine* (10th edn). Oxford: Oxford University Press, pp. 262–83.

Likierman, H. and Rachman, S. (1982). Obsessions: an experimental investigation of thought-stopping and habituation training. *Behavioural Psychotherapy* **10**, 324–38.

Lopatka, C. and Rachman, S. (1995). Perceived responsibility and compulsive checking: an experimental analysis. *Behaviour Research and Therapy* **33**, 673–84.

McLean, P. and Woody, S. (2001). *Anxiety disorders in adults.* New York: Oxford University Press.

McNally, R.J. (1994). *Panic disorder: a critical analysis.* New York: Guilford Press.

Marks, I. (1987). *Fears, phobias and rituals: panic, anxiety and their disorders.* Oxford: Oxford University Press.

Mowrer, O.H. (1939). A stimulus–response theory of anxiety. *Psychological Review* **46**, 553–65.

Mowrer, O.H. (1960). *Learning theory and behavior.* New York: Wiley.

Newth, S. and Rachman, S. (2001). The concealment of obsessions. *Behaviour Research and Therapy* **39**, 457–64.

Niler, E. and Beck, S. (1989). The relationships among guilt, dysphoria, anxiety and obsessions in a normal population. *Behaviour Research and Therapy* **27**, 213–20.

Nisbett, R. and Ross, L. (1980). *Human inference: strategies and shortcomings of social judgement.* Englewood Cliffs, NJ: Prentice-Hall.

Obsessive Compulsive Cognitions Working Group. (1997). Cognitive assessment of OCD. *Behaviour Research and Therapy* **35**, 667–81.

Obsessive Compulsive Cognitions Working Group. (2001). Development and initial validation of the obsessive beliefs questionnaire and the interpretation of intrusions inventory. *Behaviour Research and Therapy* **39**, 987–1006.

Osborn, I. (1998). *Tormenting thoughts and secret rituals.* New York: Pantheon Press.

Parkinson, L. and Rachman, S. (1980). Speed of recovery from an uncontrived stress. In S. Rachman (ed.), *Unwanted intrusive cognitions.* Oxford: Pergamon Press.

Purdon, C. (1999). Thought suppression and psychopathology. *Behaviour Research and Therapy* **37**, 1029–54.

Purdon, C. (2001). Appraisal of obsessional thought recurrences: impact on anxiety and mood state. *Behaviour Research and Therapy* **39**, 1163–81.

Purdon, C. and Clark, D.A. (1994). Obsessive intrusive thoughts in non-clinical subjects. *Behaviour Research and Therapy* **32**, 403–10.

Purdon, C. and Clark, D.A. (1999). Metacognition and obsessions. *Clinical Psychology and Psychotherapy* **6**, 102–10.

Rachman, S. (1971). Obsessional ruminations. *Behaviour Research and Therapy* **9**, 229–35.

Rachman, S. (1976a). The modification of obsessions. *Behaviour Research and Therapy* **14**, 437–43.

Rachman, S. (1976b). Obsessional-compulsive checking. *Behaviour Research and Therapy* **14**, 269–77.

Rachman, S. (1978). An anatomy of obsessions. *Behavioural Analysis and Modification* **2**, 253–78.

Rachman, S. (1983). Obstacles to the treatment of obsessions. In E.B. Foa and P.M.G. Emmelkamp (eds), *Failures in behaviour therapy*. New York: Wiley, pp. 35–57.

Rachman, S. (1993). Obsessions, responsibility, and guilt. *Behaviour Research and Therapy* **31**, 149–54.

Rachman, S. (1994). Pollution of the mind. *Behaviour Research and Therapy* **32**, 311–14.

Rachman, S. (1997a). The evolution of cognitive-behaviour therapy. In D.M. Clark and C. Fairburn (eds), *The science and practice of cognitive behaviour therapy*. Oxford: Oxford University Press, pp. 1–26.

Rachman, S. (1997b). *Anxiety*. Hove Sussex: Erlbaum.

Rachman, S. (1997c). A cognitive theory of obsessions. *Behaviour Research and Therapy* **35**, 793–802.

Rachman, S. (1998). A cognitive theory of obsessions: elaborations. *Behaviour Research and Therapy* **36**, 385–401.

Rachman, S. (2002a). A cognitive theory of compulsive checking. *Behaviour Research and Therapy* **40**, 625–40.

Rachman, S. (2002b). Compulsive checking. In R. Menzies and P. de Silva (eds), *Obsessive-compulsive disorders: theory, research and treatment*. Wiley, London, in press.

Rachman, S. and de Silva, P. (1978). Abnormal and normal obsessions. *Behaviour Research and Therapy* **16**, 233–48.

Rachman, S. and Hodgson, R. (1980). *Obsessions and compulsions*. Englewood Cliffs, NJ: Prentice-Hall.

Rachman, S. and Shafran, R. (1998). Cognitive and behavioural features of OCD. In R. Swinson, M.A. Antony, S. Rachman, and M.A. Richter (eds), *Obsessive-compulsive disorder: theory, research and treatment*. New York: Guilford Press, pp. 51–78.

Rachman, S. and Shafran, R. (1999). Cognitive distortions: thought–action fusion. *Clinical Psychology and Psychotherapy* **6**, 80–5.

Rachman, S., Shafran, R., Mitchell, D., Trant, J. and Teachman, B. (1996). How to remain neutral: an experimental analysis of neutralization. *Behaviour Research and Therapy* **34**, 889–98.

Rassin, E., Diepstraten, P., Merckelbach, H. and Muris, P. (2001). Thought–action fusion and thought suppression in OCD. *Behaviour Research and Therapy* **7**, 757–64.

Ricciardi, J.N. and McNally, R.J. (1995). Depressed mood is related to obsessions, but not to compulsions, in obsessive-compulsive disorder. *Journal of Anxiety Disorders* **9**, 249–56.

Rocca, L., Antony, M. and Swinson, R. (1998). *The expression of anger across the anxiety disorders*. Presented at the meeting of the ASSN for the Advancement of Behavior Therapy, Washington. D.C., November.

Salkovskis, P. (1985). Obsessional-compulsive problems: a cognitive-behavioural analysis. *Behaviour Research and Therapy* **23**, 571–83.

Salkovskis, P. (1996). The cognitive approach to anxiety: threat beliefs, safety-seeking behaviour, and the special case of health anxiety and obsessions. In P.M. Salkovskis (ed.), *Frontiers of cognitive therapy.* New York: Guilford Press, pp. 48–74.

Salkovskis, P. (1998). Psychological approaches to the understanding of obsessional problems, in *Obsessive Compulsive Disorder: Theory, Research Treatment,* edited R. Swinson, M. Antony, S. Rachman and M. Richter. Guilford Press, New York, pp. 33–50.

Salkovskis, P. (1999). Understanding and treating obsessive compulsive disorder. *Behaviour Research and Therapy* **37**, 529–52.

Salkovskis, P. and Campbell, P. (1994). Thought suppression induces intrusion in naturally occurring negative intrusive thoughts. *Behaviour Research and Therapy* **32**, 1–8.

Salkovsksis, P.M. and Harrison, J. (1984). Abnormal and normal obsessions: a replication. *Behaviour Research and Therapy* **22**, 549–52.

Salkovskis, P. and Kirk, J. (1997). Obsessive-compulsive disorder. In D.M. Clark and C. Fairburn (eds), *The science and practice of cognitive behaviour therapy.* Oxford: Oxford University Press, pp. 179–208.

Schwartz, J. (1996). *Brain lock.* New York: Harper Collins.

Shafran, R. (1997). The manipulation of responsibility in OCD. *British Journal of Clinical Psychology* **36**, 397–408.

Shafran, R. and Mansell, W. (2001). Perfectionism and psychopathology. *Clinical Psychology Review* **21**, 879–906.

Shafran, R., Thordarson, D.S. and Rachman, S. (1996). Thought–action fusion in obsessive-compulsive disorder. *Journal of Anxiety Disorders* **10**, 379–91.

Steketee, G. (1994). *Treatment of obsessive-compulsive disorder.* New York: Guilford Press.

Stein, M., Forde, D., Anderson, G. and Walker, J. (1997). Obsessive compulsive disorder in the community: an epidemiological survey with clinical reappraisal. *American Journal of Psychiatry* **154**, 1120–6.

Stern, R.S., Lipsedge, M. and Marks, I. (1973). Obsessional ruminations: a controlled trial of a thought-stopping technique. *Behaviour Research and Therapy* **11**, 659–62.

Teasdale, J. (1999). Emotional processing, three modes of mind and the prevention of relapse in depression. *Behaviour Research and Therapy* **37**, 553–77.

Thordarson, D. (2001). The significance of obsessions. Ph.D. thesis, University of Britiish Columbia.

Tversky, A. and Kahneman, D. (1974). Judgment under uncertainty: heuristics and biases. *Science* **185**, 1124–31.

Van Oppen, P. and Arntz, A. (1994). Cognitive therapy for obsessive compulsive disorder. *Behaviour Research and Therapy* **32**, 79–87.

Van Oppen, P. and Emmelkamp, P. (2000). Issues in cognitive treatment of obsessive-compulsive disorder. In W. Goodman, M. Rudorfer, and J. Maser (eds), *Obsessive compulsive disorder: contemporary issues in treatment.* Hillsdale, New Jersey: Erlbaum, pp. 117–32.

Welkowitz, L., Struening, E., Pitman, J., Guardino, M. and Welkowitz, J. (2000). Obsessive compulsive disorder and co-morbid anxiety problems in a national anxiety screening sample. *Journal of Anxiety Disorders* **14**, 471–82.

Wegner, D.M. and Pennebaker, J.W. (Ed.) (1993). *Handbook of mental control*. Englewood Cliffs, NJ: Prentice-Hall.

Zucker, B., Craske, M., Barrios, V. and Holguin, M. (2002). Thought–action fusion: can it be corrected? *Behaviour Research and Therapy* **40**, 653–5.

Index